Housi

D1136546

)2

This book is dedicated to
Nick, Annie and Drew
who gave me my wonderful life

Jean Conway

This book represents a celebration of Jean Conway's professional life as a housing practitioner, researcher and acamedic. She understood the central importance of housing in everyone's life and was committed to bringing an understanding of the housing system to as wide an audience as possible. She died of breast cancer when the manuscript was almost finished; it has been a privilege for us to complete the book for Jean.

Ian Cole, Colin Foster, Caroline Hunter and *Judy Nixon*

Housing Policy

Jean Conway

Gildredge Social Policy Series is published by:

The Gildredge Press Ltd
16 Gildredge Road
Eastbourne
East Sussex
BN21 4RL
United Kingdom

First Published 2000 by The Gildredge Press Ltd
Copyright © The Gildredge Press Ltd 2000

Cover Design: Clare Truscott
Cover Illustration: David Sim/The Organisation
Typeset by Central Southern Typesetters, Eastbourne, East Sussex
Printed and Bound in Great Britain by Creative Print and Design Wales
ISBN 0–9533571–2–0

Contents

    Outline   144
    The big picture   144
    The role of different housing markets   146
    The role of social housing   148
    The role of the state   151
    The role of housing professionals   154
    Key points   156
    Guide to further reading   157

    Sources
    List of references   158
    List of the main UK housing agencies and organizations 161
    List of abbreviations   162
    Some useful internet sites   163
    Index   172

Tables

Figures

Series introduction

Social policy in the United Kingdom has undergone major changes since the mid-1970s and particularly since the election of the first Thatcher government in 1979. The post-war consensus is long gone and far-reaching changes have been made in every area of social policy. These changes, of principle and of practice, have been guided both by ideology and by the context of a post-industrial and increasingly globalized economy. The emergence of New Labour has added a new and still developing dimension of change.

The growing number of students of social policy, whether in higher education or in advanced level courses such as AS/A levels and GNVQs, and including those training for professional qualifications, have to make sense of this fast-changing scene, to consider the long-term effects, and to make their own judgements of the deep-rooted issues of value that are involved.

This new series of introductory textbooks is aimed specifically at these students. The books are not academic monographs but short, tightly structured texts written with both the academic student and the trainee professional in mind. All the authors are currently involved in teaching and in policy development.

The books are designed to be aids to learning. Each book opens with a brief history and background to its policy area, followed by a review of current provision, and concludes with a discussion of future issues and possible developments. They thus present students with a concise, clear and up-to-date summary of what they need to know and understand in each area of social policy.

NOTE ON REFERENCING

This is an introductory textbook for students beginning their study of housing policy as part of an undergraduate degree or a professional or vocational qualification. It is intended to guide readers to the main issues and questions in the field, and to provide pointers to further reading or other avenues which they may wish to follow up to develop their knowledge or extend their studies. We have therefore avoided the extensive use of references to back up arguments or support empirical statements, as would normally be found in more traditional academic books. Instead, referencing is used to guide the reader to further sources which they may wish to investigate to find out more about the issues raised and questions asked in the text. There is also a short guide to further reading at the end of each chapter, together with a list of websites and other sources of information at the end of the book.

Perspectives on housing

Outline

Chapter 1 considers housing from a number of different perspectives and introduces the inherent complexity and variety in the subject, which the rest of the book follows up in greater depth. All of these perspectives are the subject of analysis by a wide range of disciplines – economists, sociologists, social policy and political analysts, planners, architects, lawyers, environmental health officers, building and engineering experts, historians and environmentalists. Housing professionals have to try to understand their field in all these ways. This makes housing both a fascinating and a challenging area of study. It may also inhibit the recognition of housing as a field of work and study in its own right.

A BASIC NEED

Shelter, water and food are generally accepted as the basic needs of life. Housing is a fundamental need; it provides shelter and also gives access to a decent water supply. In many circumstances it also affects your ability to get an adequate food supply. However, housing issues and housing policy in the UK today have a low profile, both in the minds of the general public and on the political agenda. Housing is not generally thought of as an area of professional activity – the idea of housing as a subject of academic study is often greeted with genuine surprise.

This was not always the case. In the late nineteenth century, following spectacular urban growth, poor housing conditions were identified as the root of disease, a poor quality workforce and army, and moral malaise; and substantial amounts of new building were undertaken. In the years after the Second World War, the shortage of housing again raised the issue. Since then, however, improvements in general housing conditions have brought complacency about housing which has taken it off the public agenda. Other areas of public policy take decent housing for granted. This was illustrated when the move towards care in the community in the late 1980s assumed that everyone had a suitable home in the community in which to receive their care. Professionals working in the health, welfare and criminal fields are aware of the housing needs of their clients but often assume that there is a housing safety net, and it is simply a matter of getting the local council to provide a decent place to live. Politicians find that a very high proportion of their surgery time concerns individuals' housing problems, yet they fail to raise the profile of housing in the broader political debate.

This lack of a clear public and policy focus on housing partly reflects the fact that most people in this country are well housed, and don't anticipate having to turn to public services (as they may for health or education). The lack of a clear policy also reflects the inherent complexity of the housing issue. It is an economic and financial issue, a social policy issue, and it relates to the environment and communities, and to the shape of our cities and towns. A unified policy must take account of all of these issues.

> Perceptions of housing problems vary according to the standpoint of the beholder. Different interests and perceptions generate different analyses and policy proposals.
>
> (Malpass and Murie 1999 p. 4)

HOUSING AND SOCIAL HISTORY

> History is reflected in contemporary residential patterns, forms of tenure, systems of subsidy and political attitudes.
>
> (Lund 1996 p. ix)

Housing is a durable commodity and we can only appreciate the current situation by reference to the past.

- One-third of the current housing stock is more than 60 years old, while new building adds less than 1% to it each year.
- The origins of state intervention in housing were a concern with health and the quality of the workforce, together with fear of social unrest.
- There was a massive shift in tenure patterns in the twentieth century, from predominantly private renting to owner occupation.
- Social renting (local authority and Registered Social Landlords – RSLs – is developing into a residual sector. See Chapter 4 for a discussion of residualization.

- A century of state intervention in housing has failed to break the link between poverty and poor housing.
- Substantial redevelopment took place in the 1960s and 1970s, including the building of tower blocks.

These historical constraints not only provide the framework in which current policy must operate, but may also limit the effectiveness of policies.

Housing as a health issue

Rapid urbanization in the eighteenth and nineteenth centuries resulted in appalling housing conditions for the working class. This did not trouble employers and politicians until the nineteenth-century cholera epidemics threatened the well housed as well as the poor. It was gradually recognized that insanitary housing created a health risk to all, resulted in a poor quality and weak workforce, and could lead to social unrest. In spite of fierce resistance to the idea of state intervention in the private market, public concern led to attempts to clear up the worst areas.

The main focus of interest was the physical condition of existing housing. Concern over broader housing issues such as overcrowding and shortage only emerged later. However, for most of the twentieth century there was a gradual and slow emergence of broader housing concerns such as access and cost. It was not until 1951, however, that the Ministry of Housing and Local Government were created and housing was established as an area of public policy in its own right.

Shifting tenure patterns

Before the First World War, about 10% of housing was owner occupied and 90% was rented. Charitable trusts and associations developed to provide 'model dwellings', but made a very small contribution. The First World War changed attitudes to state intervention and set the scene for local councils to play a key role.

Both world wars were followed by major tenure shifts, with large-scale slum clearance (which predominantly affected private rented housing) and major council building programmes followed by booms in private building for ownership.

Policy since the 1960s

Since the 1960s, there has been broad agreement between major political parties that, following slum clearance, the role of council housing would gradually be reduced, and owner occupation would become the dominant tenure. This accelerated during the 1980s.

Practitioners and policy makers today are faced with a tenure pattern developed over the last century and a half, and a housing stock much of which was built decades ago to the prevailing standards and expectations. These historical constraints limit the effectiveness of any policy changes. The history of intervention in housing is a key element of social history, and raises the question of the effectiveness of the state. Although the chronic housing conditions of the nineteenth century have been dealt with, many people still live in homes which are inadequate and statutorily unfit, or do not have access to a secure home at all. The poorest people still live in the poorest housing. Chapter 2 examines these historical trends in greater detail and traces the development of each housing tenure.

HOUSING AND ECONOMICS

There has been a growing recognition of the significant role which housing plays in the wider economy.

- Housing is a major fixed asset and there are considerable flows of money into and out of the sector.
- The house price increases of the late 1980s fuelled consumption, a major factor in the general inflationary boom.
- The house price slump in the early 1990s exacerbated and prolonged the economic recession, partly through high unemployment in the construction sector.
- With increasing levels of home ownership, any instability in the housing market has a major effect on the general economy.
- The cost of housing represents a major expenditure in most household budgets – governing the availability of income to spend on other goods.
- Housing is a major investment constituting about 40% of personal wealth of private individuals.

The amount of money borrowed by owner-occupiers is more than half the total Gross Domestic Product (GDP) of the UK. The market value of owner-occupied housing stock is one-and-a-half times the value of GDP. It is not surprising, therefore, that changes in the financial fortunes of the housing market have a major impact on the whole economy.

The long-term increase in owner occupation was boosted in th 1980s by three factors:

- the introduction of the right to buy for council tenants
- a rise in post-tax incomes
- easier access to mortgages following the financial deregulatio of building societies and banks.

During the late 1980s, the housing boom led to a marked increas in spending which was a major factor in the general inflationar boom. The consequences were far reaching: higher wages, los competitiveness, high interest rates, widening regiona imbalances in house prices and restricted geographical mobilit of labour.

In the first half of the 1990s, the fall in house prices and th resulting negative equity (where the value of the property fall below the amount borrowed) led to a general lack of confidenc and a reduction in new building. This exacerbated and prolonge the recession in the economy as a whole. One key factor is the rol of employment in the construction industry and relate industries. Since the late 1980s, half a million constructio workers have lost their jobs, amounting to over one-fifth of th increase in unemployment. Construction has a significant effec on activities such as architecture and surveying, supply o building materials and household goods, and buying and sellin houses. It is estimated that for every extra person employed ir construction, one extra job is created elsewhere in the economy Investment in housing is a key factor in employment levels.

The effects of housing boom and bust are far reachin throughout the economy as a whole. The volatility of the housin market aggravates the instability in the general economy anc disrupts attempts to generate steady economic growth. The UK housing market fluctuates more sharply than most othei advanced economies. In addition, moves to a more flexible labou market, such as increased unemployment and casualization, and reduced overtime, have a direct effect on the housing security of homeowners.

HOUSING AND FINANCE

By all accounts, the current housing finance system is both inefficient and unfair. It can also be viewed as plainly irrational.
(Gibbs and Munro 1991)

Housing finance is complex and results from a multitude of *ad hoc* changes over the years. Yet government decisions about how housing is paid for directly affect the housing options and choices available, and underpin much of the public debate about housing.

- There is a wide range of government measures which affect the price of housing in all tenures, and influence both the cost of supplying housing and the cost to the occupier.
- The total value of government subsidies to housing has been rising, but has shifted from subsidizing the cost of supplying homes towards subsidizing the cost of renting or buying for the consumer.
- Very few local authorities now receive any subsidy; most contribute towards the cost of Housing Benefit for their tenants.
- The increase in rents has raised concerns about affordability and provides disincentives for those on benefit to work.
- The current system of housing finance is wasteful and inequitable and needs major reform.

Very few people can claim to understand fully the way housing is financed. The system today has emerged as a series of often unconnected steps, influenced by factors other than housing policy such as the taxation and social security systems and public sector borrowing levels. Housing finance is constantly changing.

The way housing is financed results from a series of government measures which affect the price of housing. Some are geared to the suppliers of housing to reduce the cost of providing property or encourage investment, while other measures are geared to consumers to reduce their costs. Taken together, these measures produce massive flows of money. In spite of government rhetoric about cutting public expenditure, the aggregate cost of housing policies rose steadily throughout the twentieth century, particularly in the 1980s and 1990s, accentuating the importance of housing in the general economy.

The relationships between the value of these subsidies has altered greatly over time, especially in the 1980s and 1990s. The key trend has been the shift from subsidizing the *production of housing* (through subsidies to local authorities and housing associations and other RSLs for building houses) to subsidizing the *cost of using housing* (through both Housing Benefit to tenants and mortgage interest tax relief to owner-occupiers). This is often referred to as moving from 'bricks and mortar' to 'consumption' subsidies.

Housing Benefit is now the single largest item of spending on housing.

The current package of housing finance is inefficient and wasteful and produces gross inequalities between and within tenures. It results in housing shortages, poor quality accommodation, polarization between tenures, unaffordable housing and poverty traps. There have been several attempts to come up with proposals for reform across all tenures, which could achieve a fairer and less chaotic result. Most notable among these was the report on the inquiry by a National Federation of Housing Associations (NFHA) committee chaired by the Duke of Edinburgh in the mid-1980s, and a subsequent second report (NFHA 1985/1991). However, the system is so complex and so deeply embedded in all aspects of both national and household expectations that no government is seriously committed to embarking on comprehensive change. We are stuck with an arbitrary system of housing finance, which has developed over time. Housing finance is discussed in more detail in Chapter 2 and the implications for household housing costs are discussed in Chapter 4.

HOUSING AND POLITICS

The importance of housing to each individual and the scale of the financial interests involved make it a highly political issue.

- Political ideologies, particularly the differing views on the role of the state versus the market, have always shaped housing policies.
- Major interest groups involved in housing – such as the building industry, banks and building societies, the financial markets and landowners – have always tried to influence policy making in their own interests.
- The role of local authorities has been controversial. The 1980s Conservative governments saw them as a threat to both the power of central government and the freedom of consumers.
- There is some evidence that housing experiences can affect individual voting behaviour.
- Housing was a key issue in elections in the past, but has recently slipped off the political agenda.

The development of housing policies can be traced through the evolution of political ideologies. *Laissez-faire* economics, social reformism, Marxist political economy and the New Right movement have in turn influenced the perception of housing problems and the approach to dealing with them. The concept of housing as a basic social good, which the state should ensure, emerged in the early twentieth century, as social reformism took over from *laissez-faire* economics. In the 1980s and 1990s the New Right abandoned this idea and housing was again seen as a matter of individual responsibility, best provided by the market.

Interest groups

The key players in housing include landowners, the construction industry, banks, building societies, the financial markets and homeowners, as well as a range of public and other agencies. While none of these has had a consistent influence on housing policy, there have been many examples of such interests influencing the direction of change. For example, the government support of high-rise building in the 1950s and 1960s reflected the need of the building industry at the time to use industrialized building techniques. In the late 1970s, the house purchase lending markets were concerned at the slow-down in the expansion of owner occupation, as the shift from private renting reached its limit; the search for other ways of boosting the growth in owner occupation led to the right to buy for council tenants.

On the whole, tenants have not been able to operate as an effective interest group, but there have been a few notable examples (see p. 135), and the influence of homeowners has been exercised only inadvertently, if at all.

The role of local authorities

State intervention in housing has mainly been through local authorities, and they have become landlords with control over a significant proportion of the nation's households. The Conservative governments of the 1980s saw the power of local authorities as a threat to central government, particularly when many were controlled by Labour administrations. Central government increasingly took powers away from local authorities in the 1980s and 1990s, and established a network of political and financial constraints on them.

Housing and elections

There has been conflicting evidence about whether tenure is now a more important determinant of voting behaviour than class.

The Conservative governments of the 1980s believed that tenants who bought their council homes would shift their allegiance from Labour to Conservative and break the block of Labour voters on council estates.

For much of the twentieth century there was broad political consensus about the need for slum clearance and new council building, with housing featuring as a key election issue. However, as the most obvious housing problems have been dealt with and the majority of households are now well-housed owners, housing has slipped off the political agenda. The marginal seats in the 1997 election had high proportions of owner-occupiers and none of the main parties focused on housing. This was in spite of the high proportion of housing problems brought to MPs and local councillors by their constituents. In its campaign to raise the profile of housing, the Chartered Institute of Housing has highlighted the importance of housing for other services such as health, education and the criminal justice system.

HOUSING AND LAW

No social policy can be implemented without recourse to the law. The law interacts with housing in the following ways:

- It defines the relationships between the different owners and occupiers of land, e.g. the rights of tenants and mortgagors.
- Policy changes – e.g. the introduction of standards for housing – are implemented through statutes, which are then interpreted by the courts.
- When new rights are given to tenants – e.g. of security of tenure – these are done through statutes, which again will be subject to interpretation.
- The courts have a role in overseeing the conduct of public bodies, such as local authorities.

Law is a mixture of rules developed by the courts over many centuries, which are set through case law and statutes passed by Parliament. The basic framework of the nineteenth century gave very few rights to tenants and imposed few standards on landlords. The relationships were primarily governed by contract, with little control over the terms and conditions.

The increasing intervention of the state during the twentieth century saw a raft of housing statutes and other measures which control the relationships between landlords and tenants, and between lenders and borrowers. They also impose standards on landlords and duties on local authorities to enforce those standards and to provide housing for the homeless. Where duties are imposed on local authorities, or they are given discretionary powers, the courts have a role in ensuring that those duties and powers are exercised fairly, and challenges can be made (e.g. to allocation decisions) where they are not.

As greater legal controls are imposed, those who gain rights inevitably seek to exercise them, while those on whom they are imposed seek to avoid them. A good example of this arose during the 1970s and 1980s when private sector landlords sought to avoid granting tenancies under the Rent Act 1977, which gave tenants security of tenure and the right to a fair rent. They did this by the use of licence agreements, which fell outside the Act. These were challenged by tenants through the courts, first unsuccessfully, but ultimately with success in the House of Lords.

Housing policy will generally be implemented through the imposition or alteration of legally enforceable rules and regulations, so it is important to understand how the law affects whether a policy will be successful.

HOUSE BUILDING AND MAINTENANCE

From a technical perspective, housing is about the stock of dwellings.

- While there is no longer a massive national shortage of houses, there are serious shortages in some areas, particularly of homes to rent for those who cannot buy.
- In spite of huge slum clearance programmes in the past, much current housing is in very poor condition.
- House building and repairs are a major component of the construction industry, and the health of the construction industry is at the heart of the health of the economy (see p. 60).

After the Second World War, great attention was paid to housing shortages. Political parties vied with each other to build more new homes and the building boom gradually reduced the level of shortages. By the late 1970s it could be argued that there was no longer a national shortage of homes, although there were still shortages in some areas. However, recent debate about housing shortages has taken into account not just the crude numbers of households and dwellings but also whether those in need have access to those homes, which requires consideration of where the homes are situated. Consideration must also be given to the standard of the homes provided.

In spite of the slum clearance programmes, today over 1.5 million homes are unfit and one in five requires over £1,000 of urgent repairs. In the late 1960s there was a decisive policy shift away from demolishing houses towards renovating them. At the current low rate of demolition, every new home will have to last 3,500 years. However, the level of renovation and improvement fell in the 1980s and 1990s, and the condition of much of the housing stock is deteriorating. A failure to deal with the problem will bring greater costs in the longer term, including the costs of treating the poor health of those living in inadequate homes and of a return to major demolition programmes. This applies to both local authority and owner-occupied housing.

The low level of both new building and renovation has badly affected the construction industry. This has repercussions on the economy as a whole with high unemployment and reduced demand for building materials and household goods.

HOUSING AND HEALTH

There has always been an important connection between housing and health.

- Housing policy emerged out of environmental health activity to deal with urban slums.
- Environmental health is still an important element in housing work, especially in tackling poor conditions in the private sector.
- Both environmental health and housing should play a key role in the new approach to public health.

Decent housing was recognized as essential to good health more than a century ago, and the concern about ill-health led to the development of housing policy. As slum clearance and new build programmes brought significant housing improvements, and the focus of health services shifted away from environmental effects towards a medical approach, housing and health policies gradually separated. However, there is now a renewed interest from both sides in the links between housing and health. Poor housing conditions such as damp, mould, condensation and cold persist and can cause poor health.

Poor housing conditions result in additional costs for health and social care services. The NHS has to spend money treating housing-related illnesses such as asthma, heart and respiratory problems; the increasing incidence of TB; accidents in the home and house fires. The economy as a whole bears the cost of productivity lost through illness. Demands on social care agencies are increased by the mental stress associated with inadequate housing and care programmes are less effective where housing is unsuitable. The connection between housing, health and community care programmes is considered further in Chapter 5.

HOUSING, PLANNING AND THE ENVIRONMENT

Housing has a major impact on the environment, some aspects of which are controlled through the planning system.

- Homes produce 25% of CO_2 emissions in the UK, consume significant amounts of energy and water resources and produce large amounts of waste.
- House building and repairs use large amounts of building materials, many of which are natural non-renewable resources or toxic.
- New building uses up large amounts of land and there is growing pressure on rural and greenbelt areas.
- The standard of many new houses has fallen, yet there is greater need for good quality adaptable homes to meet a wide range of mobility needs.
- Planning has a key role in the development of housing.
- Planning considerations affect the type of housing which is built, its location and its cost.

The planning system helps resolve the conflicting demands on land use. The amount and location of land which the planning system makes available affects its price, and land costs can be as much as 40% of the price of a new house in high pressure areas. The planning system also affects the density of development, what sort of homes are built, the local environment and the long-term environmental impact of development. These issues are considered further in Chapter 3.

Housing has a major and ongoing impact on the environment. A serious attempt to make housing more environmentally sensitive could have a significant effect on the UK's achievement of the 'Agenda for the 21st century' agreed at the 1992 Earth Summit in Rio de Janeiro. Chapter 3 discusses sustainable housing and the environment in more detail.

HOUSING AND SOCIOLOGY

Housing policies must take account of the wider social context in which housing is set. Sociology makes an important contribution to housing, notably through the light which it sheds on:

- the causes of inequality and the ways in which class, status, gender and race shape housing provision
- the ideologies and roles of the various housing interest groups.

Housing not only reflects social inequalities but sustains and exacerbates them. A sociological perspective has shed light on the processes by which divisions in society are established and maintained, and on the role played by the various managers of the housing process such as politicians and private and public sector professionals as well as those working in local and central government. Where you live affects your prospects of health, education, jobs, support and security. Inequalities in the housing system are discussed in Chapter 4.

HOUSING AND SOCIAL EXCLUSION

The Labour government elected in 1997 put a major focus on linking housing to broader strategies to combat social exclusion, specifically through the Social Exclusion Unit. The unit was established in 1997 to devise and implement policies to prevent social exclusion, and describes social exclusion as:

> a shorthand label for what can happen when individuals or areas suffer from a combination of linked problems such as unemployment, poor skills, low incomes, poor housing, high crime environment, bad health and family breakdown
>
> (Social Exclusion Unit 1998)

Housing is central to this work.

- Children in poor and overcrowded homes are at a disadvantage in education.
- Poor housing harbours crime and anti-social behaviour.
- The cost and location of housing affects incentives and opportunities to get work.

Education

The condition of your home, and its location and cost, can limit your wider life chances. Children's development and education require a suitable home environment, which provides security, stability and space. Children living in temporary accommodation, such as bed and breakfast hotels, are particularly badly affected and have been shown to suffer from slow development, and behavioural and psychological problems. Poor housing can hinder the full development of a child's potential and lead to educational disadvantage.

Crime

The level of crime, particularly burglary and robbery, is higher than average in some social housing estates. Both the incidence and the fear of crime restrict people's movement, stigmatize estates and make people less caring about their environment generally. Councils spend a lot of money dealing with the results of burglaries and vandalism on estates and there are huge costs for the police and criminal justice system. Design changes, security measures and housing management initiatives can be effective in reducing the level of crime on estates.

Employment

Where you live affects your access to jobs, and housing needs to be available and affordable close to employment markets. Living in insecure housing, and homelessness in particular, make it very difficult to find and keep a job. The high rent strategy (see p. 83) has had a major effect on work incentives, because many jobs do not pay well enough to cover the rent when Housing Benefit is lost, and tenants become stuck in the 'poverty trap'. There have been a number of projects which combine housing renovation work with job training for local unemployed people, and the government has linked together the home insulation programme and youth training.

Responses to social exclusion

The essential relationships between housing and other services have increasingly been recognized in government regeneration programmes. The City Challenge Programme and Single Regeneration Budget are aimed at comprehensive area strategies including physical, economic and social measures, although the funds for these schemes are severely limited. Housing agencies are also getting involved in anti-poverty strategies and projects to tackle social exclusion, especially through the New Deal for Communities programme and the work of the Social Exclusion Unit. These innovations are discussed in Chapter 3.

There is a concentration of poverty on certain housing estates following the residualization of social housing. See Chapter 4 for a discussion of residualization. Attempts to tackle social exclusion must include housing programmes to be effective. The lack of investment in housing over the last few decades of the twentieth century increased demands on a range of other services and is costly both to those who are not decently housed and to the economy as a whole.

THE CONTENT AND STRUCTURE OF THIS BOOK

This book looks at all the different aspects of housing and tries to relate housing policy and practice to the range of other public services and the work of other professions. In order to keep the book within a manageable length, the focus is primarily on England and Wales, although specific consideration is given to structures in Scotland and Northern Ireland in Chapter 2. A greater understanding of housing by related professionals would help to foster improved working links. It is hoped that this book will make a small contribution to this.

This book is not organized according to particular housing policy problems and responses, but rather the chapters are thematic, illustrating the interaction between different policies. Therefore some issues find a place in more than one chapter – e.g. homelessness emerges as an issue in the context of housing as home (Chapter 4), housing as a service (Chapter 6) and housing, health and social care (Chapter 5). While each chapter may be considered individually, it is hoped that readers will consider the book as a whole. The multi-faceted nature of housing illustrated in this opening chapter does not allow for simple solutions to problems. Rather housing must be thought of holistically and as reflecting the interdependence of different topics.

The one exception to the broad, thematic approach is Chapter 5, which focuses on one major perspective on housing – health and social care. This topic has been selected for more detailed analysis since it demonstrates how the increasing concentration of vulnerable people in social housing brings new demands.

Highlighting the fundamental links between housing and other aspects of social welfare also demonstrates the need for improved inter-agency collaboration and the development of more effective working relationships between agencies and professions.

Finally, Chapter 7 looks to the future and outlines likely shifts in patterns of tenure, and the prospects for housing policy development in the twenty-first century.

KEY POINTS

- Housing can be viewed from a number of perspectives, each shedding light on a different aspect of the topic. A wide range of subjects and specialisms contributes to an understanding of housing.
- Housing is basic to many aspects of social welfare. Recognition of the essential links between housing and other areas of social policy requires closer working relationships between agencies and professional groups.
- There was a fragmentation and proliferation of agencies involved in all aspects of social welfare provision in the 1990s, with greater administrative complexity.

GUIDE TO FURTHER READING

For a fuller analysis of British housing policy and practice as implemented at different levels of government see:

Malpass, P. and Murie, A. (1999) *Housing Policy and Practice.* Fifth edition. London: Macmillan.

Housing as history: the development of policy, tenure and finance

Outline

This chapter looks at the development of housing policy from the mid-nineteenth century to the present day. The first section provides a brief history of housing development, and shows how this led to the housing stock of today. The second section traces the historical development of each main housing tenure in turn. The shifting balance between tenures is analysed, together with an account of the recent breakdown in the established consensus about the appropriate role of local authority housing.

The historical trends are underpinned by developments in housing finance. The section on finance outlines the broad flows of money within the housing system and highlights the inherent imbalance in the way housing money is used and the detrimental effects on the wider economy. The role of building societies is also considered, as they are the main source of finance for the dominant tenure. Finally the chapter contrasts housing policies and practices in England, N. Ireland, Scotland and Wales.

TODAY'S HOUSING STOCK: THE LEGACY OF THE PAST

The current housing stock is a result of policies implemented over the last century and a half. This section considers:

- the nineteenth-century origins of state intervention
- the inter-war boom and the development of council housing
- the post-war rise and fall in building and clearance
- continuity and change in the 1980s and 1990s.

The nineteenth-century origins of state intervention

Just under a quarter of the existing housing in Great Britain was built before the First World War, a similar proportion was built between the world wars, 24% was built in the period between 1945 and 1965, and about a third of the stock has been completed since then. These statistics show how our present housing system inevitably bears the imprint of past policies and developments.

Until the mid-nineteenth century, housing was a private affair, of no concern to the state. Only the church and private charities made some limited provision for the poor or destitute. The history of state housing policy begins about 150 years ago, and charts the gradual intervention of the state in the private market, both indirectly through controls on the activities of private owners and directly through state provision of homes. As with other areas of social policy, it was the industrial revolution and the expansion of cities which prompted state intervention.

During the industrial revolution, the rural population migrated to the towns and cities, and private housing developers responded by providing rented housing at the price people could afford. This took the form of back-to-back rows, cellars, huddled courts and tenement blocks. This housing was inevitably of extremely poor quality, with virtually no provision of water or waste disposal, and massively over-occupied.

Disease was rife, but as long as it was confined to the working classes it raised no wider concern. However, in 1832 and 1849 there were major cholera epidemics. Whereas typhus had killed the sickly, the undernourished and the poor; cholera affected everyone – including the middle classes. These epidemics therefore led to early attempts to clear up the worst areas of the towns. These attempts were short lived – the epidemics lasted about two years and when the disease declined, so did efforts to improve conditions. The rural poor also lived in appalling hovels, but these were less of a direct health threat to the rest of society.

A number of factors were important in the gradual introduction of state intervention in housing. The way in which cholera spreads was only fully understood in 1849, when it was proved that it was waterborne, and therefore the provision of clean water in cities became crucial. There was also a gradual recognition that the poor conditions of the working classes could threaten society more profoundly: the productivity of the workforce was affected by poor health, there was a growing concern that poor housing conditions could lead to social unrest, and a high proportion of army recruits were found to be medically unfit for military service, thus jeopardizing the defence of the empire. A prerequisite for state intervention on any scale was the existence of local administrative structures capable of enforcing central government policy. Elected local councils were first set up in 1835, but it was not until the 1870s that a coherent and uniform structure of local government was established.

The first piece of legislation recognizing that the state should take some responsibility for the welfare of the community was introduced in the 1840s, beginning a series of Public Health and Housing Acts. These initially focused on forcing landlords to improve their housing, starting with the provision of sewerage and water, then providing minimum standards for new houses. Later came local authority powers to close or demolish insanitary houses, followed in 1875 by powers to clear whole areas of poor housing. It was not until the 1890 Housing of the Working Classes Act that local authorities were given powers to provide housing themselves, but this did not initially result in much new provision. Up to 1914 local authorities built only about 20,000 houses.

Nineteenth-century legislation emphasized clearing the worst housing rather than replacing it. Most inner city clearance was carried out under local Acts of Parliament for civic improvements such as railway termini. More houses were demolished than built to replace them, bringing more crowding and higher rents for the displaced poor. The early housing charities and associations provided decent housing for the respectable working classes, but their reforms contributed to housing problems by evicting the 'less respectable' or 'immoral' tenants, who did not live up to the housekeeping, financial and sobriety standards expected. There was no concern about the fate of those evicted.

The nineteenth-century housing and public health legislation had little impact and few local authorities used their powers. They did not have a duty to respond, nor did they have the administrative structures to carry out an active role. There was deep-seated resistance to the idea of intervening in a free market, not least because often the elected council members were themselves the landlords who would have to foot the bill.

At the beginning of the twentieth century, a private building boom catered for those sections of the urban working population which had rising wages. Building was still concentrated in the inner cities, because living outside the centre was limited by the high cost of travel and the length of the working day. Thus the basic pattern of dense city development continued, with minimal attempts to alleviate the worst conditions.

The inter-war boom and the development of council housing

The First World War was a major turning point in the history of housing policy. New house building virtually stopped during the war but the number of households rose steeply, leading to large housing shortages. The massive increase in the role and machinery of the state during the war, coupled with huge rises in taxation, gave the government unprecedented powers over the market and the economy. The fear of social unrest was reinforced by the revolutions in central Europe and the discontent of returning war heroes. New working-class organizations developed further, including the Working Men's National Housing Council and the Labour Party, and housing became a key political issue. Coupled with the reluctant recognition that the private housing market was unable to supply enough houses to meet chronic shortages, in reasonable conditions at rents which the working classes could afford, the state was forced to accept a new responsibility to intervene.

Following a series of rent strikes, rent control was introduced in 1915. This was seen as a temporary war-time measure, but the shortage of housing after the war made it impossible to lift the controls. Direct subsidy to landlords was unacceptable to the electorate. The government reluctantly acknowledged that local authorities, already responsible for local services, were the most appropriate bodies to provide new housing with subsidies.

A series of Acts heralding an active housing role for local authorities began with the 1919 Housing and Town Planning Act, introduced by a Liberal government. This gave authorities clear new responsibilities, requiring them to produce a survey of the housing needs of their area and make plans for the provision of housing. They were given an open-ended exchequer subsidy on the cost of new houses in excess of 1-penny rate fund contributions. The age of mass local authority house building began and 170,000 dwellings were built in the two years after 1919.

However, costs proved high, reflecting a large increase in the costs of materials after the war as well as the high standards of the properties built, incorporating generous space standards and decent cooking and heating facilities. In 1923, under the Conservative government, the subsidy system was replaced by a less generous fixed subsidy, but the succeeding Labour government's 1924 Housing (Financial Provisions) Act quickly restored an active role for local authority building, with higher levels of fixed subsidy. This firmly established local authority housing and exchequer subsidy as long-term features of housing policy in Britain, a trend continuing until the early 1980s.

From the mid-1920s, new building for both landlords and

owner-occupiers began to rise, reaching a boom in the middle and late 1930s. (Indeed, this peak of private house building has not been matched since.) The building land available increased as a result of improvements in public transport to the suburbs and the absence of strict land-use controls. This was coupled with a fall in the cost of building materials and wages. Private speculative builders were able to provide houses at prices which could be afforded by the emerging lower middle classes in secure jobs in the expanding sectors of banking, insurance and public administration. They were able to buy houses with newly available fixed mortgages from the building societies. There was a rapid expansion of suburban housing estates around most cities, especially London.

With the severe post-war housing shortages, attention had focused on new building, away from public health action on poor quality existing housing. Slum clearance was at a very low level throughout the 1920s, as the building boom gradually reduced the housing shortages. Attention subsequently turned to the condition of the housing stock. A new slum clearance drive, signalled by Housing Acts in 1930 and 1933, focused on the lowest standard houses built before the 1870s. Local authorities were given special subsidies for building new homes for those households displaced by slum clearance, and they tended to provide large municipal estates on the edge of towns, often lacking shopping and other amenities. The inter-war building boom resulted in nearly four million new dwellings altogether, and provided a substantial legacy evident in our current housing stock.

The post-war rise and fall in building and clearance

As with the First World War, the Second World War saw a halting of new building activity and a rapidly growing number of households. However, this war also brought large-scale damage to the housing stock. Over 200,000 houses were totally destroyed and a quarter of a million were so damaged as to be uninhabitable. A further three million houses were damaged but were still inhabitable. The resulting post-war shortage of homes was estimated to be two million. There was strong public and political consensus for an active council house building programme and in the next five years, under a Labour government, over one million new homes were built, over 80% by local authorities.

As a further parallel with the inter-war years, the focus then shifted towards slum clearance and local authorities increasingly concentrated on building large new estates to replace the slums. Total post-war new building activity in all sectors, and in the level of slum clearance, peaked in the late 1960s and early 1970s. Nearly one in three homes today was built in the 25 years following the Second World War. The slum clearance programme was especially active in Scotland, and in Glasgow in particular.

By the late 1960s housing policies seemed to have been broadly successful in dealing with the worst of the housing problems. The post-war building boom had significantly reduced the housing shortage. The slum clearance programme had dealt with the most obvious areas for clearance and was increasingly criticized for causing blight and the wholesale disruption of communities. The remaining pockets of poor housing were considered less suitable for area demolition. This change of view, coupled with an economic crisis, led to a major shift away from slum clearance and replacement towards rehabilitation of older housing. The 1969 Housing Act brought new levels of grants for private owners to improve their property and introduced the idea of tackling whole areas of run-down housing, with improvements to the individual houses coupled with environmental works in the streets. Grant levels and area programmes for improvement were further enhanced in the early 1970s. This heralded an end to the major local authority new building programmes, which was virtually halted by the mid-1970s when the economic crisis led to the sharp cuts in public expenditure required by the International Monetary Fund.

The other major policy development in the 1970s was the attempt by the Conservative government to move towards market level rents in both the public and private sectors under the 1972 Housing Finance Act, by decontrolling private rents and forcing up council rents. The Act also brought in a national system of rent rebates for council tenants to replace the discretionary local schemes which councils had been able to run since the 1930s, and extended this to rent allowances for private tenants. This became the basis for the current system of Housing Benefit. However, the rent increases were extremely unpopular and the following Labour government ended the enforced rent regime in the mid-1970s. A decade later another Conservative administration was to move rents up towards a 'market' level once again.

Continuity and change in the 1980s and 1990s

The above analysis shows a large degree of consensus between the main political parties up to the end of the 1970s. The Conservative government from 1979 to 1997 brought a faster pace of change and signalled the end of this general agreement about the proper role of the state in housing provision.

The basis of the Conservative reforms was a desire to roll back the state and create opportunities for the private market and competition. This was driven by a New Right ideology, which considered housing a matter of individual choice and responsibility, with the state playing only a minimal role. Housing policy was no longer seen as an attempt to meet needs, but to reflect what the country could afford and what the market would provide. Support for home ownership was not novel or unique to this Conservative government, but the directly hostile treatment of local authorities, especially from the late 1980s, was a new development. Changes in housing policy were part of a new approach to public services in general, with the state becoming a purchaser rather than a provider, and competition between independent agencies to provide services under a contract.

Although the rhetoric was about rolling back the state and reducing expenditure, the policies in reality brought greater central government control and little reduction in the overall costs of housing policies. Many of the new programmes proved very expensive, including Housing Action Trusts, the Business Expansion Scheme for private renting, and preparations for the privatization of council estates and local authority housing management. Rent increases for council and housing association housing simply raised the amount of Housing Benefit needed to support the poorer tenants, and mortgage interest tax relief for home owners was out of control by the late 1980s. Local authorities and housing associations became more tightly controlled by central government and the Housing Corporation than ever before.

HOUSING TENURE SHIFTS

It is clear from the above overview of housing history that the pattern of tenure changed dramatically in the twentieth century, as shown in Figure 2.1.

Figure 2.1 Housing tenure in England and Wales 1914–1997

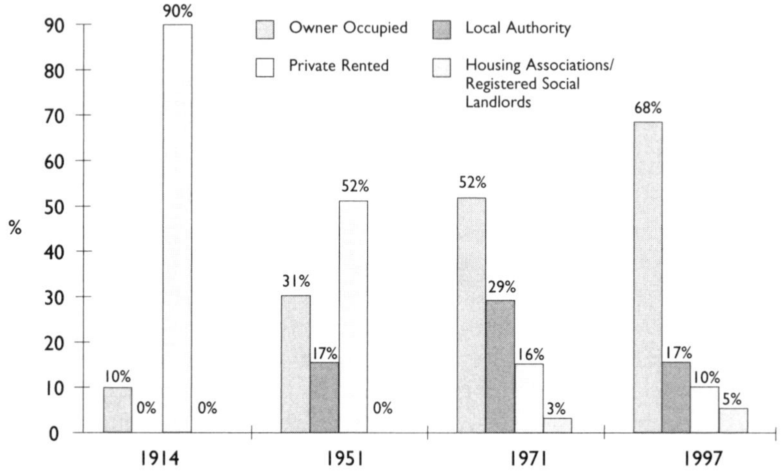

Sources: Malpass, P. and Murie, A. (1999) *Housing Policy and Practice* (Fifth edition) London: Macmillan – Table 1.1 p. 11, and Wilcox, S. (1998) *Housing Finance Review (1998/99)* York: Joseph Rowntree Foundation – Table 17b p. 93

Housing policies not only encourage or discourage new building in each tenure, but also lead to existing homes being sold from one form of ownership to another. The relentless rise of owner occupation has been matched by a parallel decline in private renting, more fitful expansion until the 1980s in council housing, and the recent emergence of the housing association sector playing a less marginal role. To explain these developments, the following analysis focuses first on the private sector and then on the public sector, highlighting the relationships between them.

The private rented sector

Until 100 years ago almost everyone except the very rich rented their home from a private landlord. The landlord was either renting out property as an investment for profit, or was the employer providing housing as part of the job. However, within a century private renting declined from housing 90% of households to about 10%. Even in the 1950s the private rented sector still housed the majority of households in Britain.

There is a number of reasons for this decline, including disincentives to renting out property and incentives for other tenures. Attempts by several governments to halt the decline have not taken effect, suggesting that the reasons are complex and fundamental to the whole housing system in Britain.

The Victorians gradually realized that private landlords could not provide sufficient decent housing at prices which the poorest households could afford. State intervention to enforce improved standards cut into profits. Prevailing low wage levels prevented landlords from simply increasing rents to compensate for increased costs. As discussed on pages 19–20, public pressures during the First World War led to the imposition of rent controls, initially expected to be a temporary measure but too politically sensitive to withdraw after the war. Landlords' profits were thus reduced. The impact of rent controls was reduced by falling general price levels between the wars, but at the outbreak of the Second World War rents were frozen and controls extended.

In this climate landlords looked to alternative uses of their capital, in terms of potential revenue returns and capital gains available. House prices are determined by the buoyancy of the private housing market, and the other form of private ownership – owner occupation – expanded rapidly between the wars to cater for the new middle classes. Rising house prices prompted many landlords to sell their houses for capital gain, which could then be invested in other, more lucrative ways.

It is sometimes assumed that rent controls are the main reason for the decline in private renting. However, most housing analysts agree that a more powerful explanation lies in the unfavourable tax and subsidy position of private renting in relation to other tenures. Unlike landlords in many other European countries, British landlords receive virtually no direct subsidy, apart from loan interest payments which are tax deductible in line with commercial business taxation. Management and maintenance costs and depreciation are borne entirely by landlords, and they are subject to capital gains tax from which owner-occupiers are exempt. In recent decades Housing Benefit paid to poorer tenants towards the rent has enabled higher rents to be charged than would otherwise be possible, but restrictions on the amount paid in benefit have kept a lid on rent levels, except at the luxury end of the market. Many landlords are reluctant to rely on tenants on Housing Benefit because of the risks of delays in payments, the bureaucracy involved and the potential impact of any cuts in the scheme, of which there have been many.

The decline in the supply of private rented housing is largely the result of the attraction of selling private rented housing into owner occupation. The other major cause of decline in the sector stems from the impact of slum clearance programmes, which have predominantly concerned private rented housing. Of the private rented housing stock in 1939, nearly 30% had been demolished by 1981. More than half of all private rented property today is owned by individuals, and the typical landlord has only a few properties.

There have been two major attempts to revive the sector, both by Conservative governments. The 1957 Rent Act removed rent and security of tenure restrictions on 10% of the stock and for all tenancies upon vacancy, and raised rent controlled levels on most of the rest. Despite the prospect of higher rents, the attraction of selling property into home ownership was still overwhelming. The reductions in security for tenants provided a new opportunity to evict tenants and sell up, so that the 1957 Rent Act in fact had the effect of hastening the decline in the sector. The Conservative government tried yet again to decontrol the sector and allow rents to rise under the 1972 Housing Finance Act, but this was repealed by the following Labour government before it achieved full impact.

More recently, the 1979–1997 Conservative governments introduced several measures to halt the decline in private renting. Rent controls were lifted and security of tenure restricted for new and renovated rented dwellings in 1980. The 1988 Housing Act introduced a new form of tenure, known as Assured Tenancies and Assured Shorthold Tenancies, which were free of rent controls, and had limited security of tenure with wider and more flexible grounds for possession for landlords. The government also strengthened tenants' protection from illegal eviction. Under the 1996 Housing Act almost all new tenancies are now Assured Shorthold, with security limited to six months and easier possession for the landlord.

In 1988 the government ended the long-term resistance to

subsidizing the sector by extending the Business Expansion Scheme (BES) to the provision of rented housing. Companies providing new or newly converted properties for renting were given a tax discount on investments and freedom from capital gains tax. The scheme resulted in a new supply of about 80,000 rented homes. It was calculated that making the same amount of money available to housing associations could have provided 80% of this output, while making them accessible to lower income tenants and capable of being retained in the rented sector for the long term (Crook *et al.* 1991). The BES scheme was ended after four years in 1993.

In 1996 a further scheme of incentives for investing in rented housing was introduced, known as Housing Investment Trusts (HITs). This also had little impact and was abandoned.

Since the late 1980s there has been an increase in the amount of private renting, from about 7% to about 10% of the housing stock. However, it is difficult to identify the extent to which this resulted from the new regime, because it coincided with the massive slump in the owner-occupied market at the end of the 1980s. With rapidly falling house prices, landlords no longer faced the traditional alternative attraction of gaining vacant possession and selling the property. In addition many owners who needed to move found they could not sell, or realized they were better off renting out their house until house prices rose again. The rise in renting of the early 1990s halted in the second half of the decade. Only longer-term trends will show whether the various measures to revive the sector have had any lasting impact.

Analysts believe that the long-term decline in private renting will not be halted while owner occupation retains tax advantages, and while landlords do not feel any security in the future for renting in the light of political uncertainties. There is increasing recognition across the political spectrum that if the private rented sector is to play a role in housing in the future, it has to be subsidized in some way to make it attractive to investors.

These disincentives to renting are reinforced on the demand side, as private renting has become less attractive than other tenures for those with any choice. However, it is accepted that the private rented sector may still have a valuable role to play in housing young, mobile adults and newly formed households. Chapter 4 discusses the types of private sector tenants and their differing needs.

Owner occupation

The fortunes of the private rented market are intricately tied up with the owner-occupied market, which became the increasingly favoured tenure for most of the twentieth century. Owner occupation has grown for a number of reasons:

- the collapse of private renting with landlords selling into ownership
- the growth of building societies and ease of gaining credit
- population and household growth
- rising real household incomes
- the popular image of ownership as providing control, autonomy and an investment
- government financial support, mainly in the form of mortgage interest tax relief (MIRAS).

Government financial support began between the wars, with local authority loans for house purchase and government cash grants for private construction, which lasted for ten years from 1923. Since the 1950s all the major parties have directly supported home ownership through a series of measures: freeing up loans from local authorities and building societies, leasehold reform, grants for improvements, giving council tenants the right to buy with discounts, various low-cost home ownership initiatives and fiscal measures relating to stamp duty, freedom from capital gains tax, VAT and MIRAS.

Tax relief on mortgage interest (known from 1983 onwards as MIRAS) was introduced as a fiscal measure rather than as a conscious policy to support home ownership. However, the cost to the Exchequer rose steeply during the house price boom of the late 1980s, and MIRAS reached a peak of £7.7 billion in 1990. From the late 1980s governments accepted the case for restricting it. The value of the tax relief was gradually cut back and MIRAS was finally phased out in the 1999 budget.

The expansion of home ownership has not been without cost in other ways. For the economy as a whole the instability in house prices in the last two decades of the twentieth century had a destabilizing effect, as explained in Chapter 1. The period of falling prices left many new owners in negative equity, where the mortgage is greater than the current value of the house, thus making it more difficult for them to sell and move. In addition, increasing numbers of owners have fallen into difficulties paying the mortgage, and arrears and repossessions have increased, as discussed in Chapter 4. This was partly as the result of the restructuring of the labour market, which brought higher levels of long-term unemployment and job insecurity.

The expansion of the sector to nearly 70% of households brought ownership to many middle- and low-income households (Forrest, Murie and Williams 1990). In addition to problems of affordability, there are increasing concerns about the future conditions of dwellings owned by those with little extra money to spend on maintenance. This is considered in Chapter 3.

The rise and fall of council housing

The emergence of state housing has to be seen in the context of trends in the private housing sector. As the brief history of housing policy above shows, towards the end of the nineteenth century it became apparent that the private rented market could not provide decent homes at prices which the working classes could afford. The fear of social unrest, rather than a concern with the welfare of the poor, prompted the gradual introduction of local authority building, later supported by state subsidies. The most effective class pressure came from the better-off, skilled workers whose labour was vital to the continued growth of the economy. Early local authority housing was therefore built to meet their needs, to high standards with relatively high rents. This is often referred to as 'general needs housing' (Kemp 1991).

The poorer working classes still relied on the private rented market. However, the growth of the slum clearance programme in the 1930s required local authorities to cater for those who had been displaced as well. House building for home ownership was taking off, giving a private alternative for the better off. The government withdrew support for general needs housing and local authorities concentrated on providing for those rehoused from the slums. The standards of council housing fell, partly to ensure that the rents would be low enough for the displaced families. The high quality council housing of the 1920s is often more popular today than the lower quality 1930s stock. By the beginning of the Second World War, the private market transition from renting to owning was well established, with the council sector providing about 10% of housing, predominantly for those not catered for by either part of the private market.

After the Second World War there was a similar pattern in the development of council housing. Chronic housing shortages required a rapid response and local authorities again built for general needs. The years between 1945 and 1955 saw the biggest local authority building boom of all time. By the mid-1950s the private market had recovered and house building for owner occupation was expanding. With pressures to reduce standards and costs in the public sector, high-rise blocks were seen as the cheapest option and subsidies were geared to the height of the block. This was accompanied by the development of system building and prefabricated techniques, which resulted in the high-rise estates of the 1960s and early 1970s. The proportion of the housing stock which was council owned continued to rise slowly, until it reached a peak of 32% in 1979.

Council housing has developed as a response to the activities of the private market (Malpass and Murie 1999). The long-term process of adjustment from private renting to owning created tensions which prompted state intervention. After both wars the private market took some time to recover, so local authorities were required to build high-standard homes for general needs. When the private market began to expand again, local authorities were confined to a more specialist role, complementary to the market rather than in competition with it. In this way council housing can be seen as a buffer during a long period of private market reorganization.

Council housing has for many years been an increasingly residual tenure, catering for the least well-off for whom the market cannot provide. While the Labour Party has always expressed more enthusiastic support for council housing than the Conservative Party, both parties have accepted the dominance of owner occupation. The Conservative government elected in 1979 actively sought to reduce the local authority sector and the 1980s witnessed the biggest tenure shifts during a single decade in history.

With the benefit of hindsight, it is easy to see that the groundwork for this attack on local authority housing had been laid much earlier. From the early 1970s council rents had been forced up through a variety of government measures, to a level where better-off tenants were paying substantial rents and were more attracted towards home ownership. The poorest tenants were helped by the national rent rebate scheme. At the same time, the relatively new blocks of council flats began to experience structural problems and the generally poor-quality estates were becoming unpopular. Traditionally low levels of maintenance, poor housing management, the lack of amenities and the growing concentration of poor households resulted in estates which were difficult to let. This undermined the image of council housing and allowed an ideological assault on the sector as a whole. Council tenants were branded as work shy, anti-social and undeserving of subsidies. Rather than being seen as the solution to housing problems, council housing was branded as part of the problem itself.

The first and most significant step in reducing the public sector was through the right to buy for council tenants, introduced in the 1980 Housing Act. Sales had been permitted as long ago as 1925, with discounts on the price introduced in 1957. Some urban Conservative housing authorities had started to sell housing on a significant scale in the late 1960s. The 1980 Act not only obliged all local authorities to sell on demand, but included a right to a local authority mortgage and brought in high levels of discounts, initially up to 50% and later rising to a maximum of 60% on houses and 70% on flats. Over one-and-three-quarter million council tenants exercised their right to buy. The council stock has been reduced by over 25%, with higher levels in the south-east of England and in Wales and lower levels in Scotland. During the early 1980s the number of dwellings sold through the right to buy exceeded the number of newly built dwellings for home ownership. The programme fuelled the expansion in owner occupation, just at the time when the scope for its growth through the transfer of the shrinking private rented sector was declining.

After the better-off tenants, who were able to buy and who lived in the most desirable homes, exercised their right to buy during the 1980s, the level of sales started to decline. The government therefore brought in a series of other measures to reduce the public sector housing stock. The 1988 Housing Act introduced several new packages for selling off local authority housing. The 1989 Housing Act backed this up by making council renting less attractive, introducing a new financial regime for local housing authorities which forced up rents, restrained spending on management and maintenance, and brought to an end the overall subsidy on council housing. Councils were left with little scope to undertake major repairs or new building. Rent surpluses were being used to cover about 30% of the cost of Housing Benefit. This is explained in more detail in the discussion of housing finance on page 39.

The 1988 Housing Act introduced Tenants' Choice and Housing Action Trusts (HATs) as mechanisms to transfer ownership of council housing estates to other landlords. Both these policies were based on a belief that tenants would leap at the opportunity to get out of council ownership, but in practice there was very little interest and Tenants' Choice was abandoned (although a similar scheme survives in Scotland and allows individual tenants to transfer to a new landlord). A small number of HATs were created but proved extremely expensive and the programme was not continued further.

'Voluntary transfers' have become the most important engine for reducing the council sector in recent years, under which local authorities can initiate the sale of all or part of their housing stock to another body with the approval of the tenants. As the financial constraints of the 1989 Housing Act have increasingly restricted their role as landlords, more and more authorities have decided to transfer their stock. The money received is used to pay off the debt on the property and any surplus can be used for local community facilities. The new landlords are often able to raise money more easily to undertake repairs. Over 60 authorities have carried out Large-Scale Voluntary Transfers (LSVTs) of their housing stock – including more than 50 which have transferred all their housing and are no longer landlords, except of temporary accommodation. Many other authorities have sold off parts of their housing stock and over a quarter of a million council homes have been transferred altogether, usually to newly established Registered Social Landlords (RSLs), discussed next.

More recently, authorities have expressed interest in setting up local housing companies – independent agencies to buy and manage the housing, with management boards composed of local authority representatives, tenants and others. Several large local authorities, especially in Scotland, are currently giving serious consideration to this option for ownership and control. However, in spite of better opportunities to get repairs done, many council tenants are reluctant to transfer, fearing rent rises and the loss of rights, and some proposals to set up companies have been rejected by the tenants.

Registered Social Landlords

The term 'Registered Social Landlords' (RSLs) was coined in the mid-1990s to refer to the sector covering housing associations, local housing companies, tenant co-operatives and other agencies potentially eligible for Housing Corporation support. RSLs currently provide just under one million dwellings, comprising 5% of the total housing stock – over a fifth of the social rented sector. RSLs are non-profit-making organizations (which are, however, allowed to make surpluses) run by voluntary management committees, with a wide variety of structures and aims. There are more than 2,200 RSLs in Britain, most of which are locally based with a handful of properties, although there is a small number of RSLs with over 10,000 dwellings, with the largest owning 40,000 properties.

The oldest housing associations were almshouse trusts and charities, some dating back to the Middle Ages, while others developed in the late nineteenth century to house older people and the poor. By 1914 they provided about 50,000 homes, mostly in London. Until recently housing associations had a predominantly specialized role, complementary to local authorities, catering for specific groups of people such as older people, the disabled or the mentally ill.

Local authorities had the power to give financial assistance to housing associations, but this was rarely used. The Housing Corporation was established in 1964 to supervise the activities of associations and distribute loans on a small scale. In 1967 associations were given subsidies to buy and improve existing properties in inner city areas. Some new organizations were set up specifically for this purpose, often in conjunction with area improvement programmes, and they made a significant contribution to inner city rehabilitation. The major development of the sector followed the 1974 Housing Act when a new range of capital and revenue grants was introduced for those associations which registered with the corporation, triggering a significant growth in activity.

The Conservative government elected in 1979 started to cut the housing association development programme, in line with its general approach to social renting and public sector borrowing. However, the cut in local authority housing was even greater, and housing association development exceeded council new building from the early 1980s. Housing associations' share of the total rented stock increased from 8% in 1982/83 to 20% in 1993/94. Activities were redirected towards low-cost home ownership schemes, such as shared ownership and improvement for sale.

Some tenants were given the right to buy, and this was extended in 1996 to almost all association tenants, with the exception of those in rural areas. Grants were also introduced to help tenants buy their current or another private home.

The 1988 Housing Act redefined housing associations as part of the 'independent' rather than the public rented sector, and radically altered the financial structure. Central government grants for development were cut and associations were required to make up any difference through private loans. Higher rents were needed to repay the loans, and new tenants became assured tenants with decontrolled rents. Associations were seen as a 'quasi private' alternative to local authorities.

In the last few years of the twentieth century, RSLs became expected to take on the role of local authorities in housing local people in need, with an increasing emphasis on homeless families. Many local authorities, unable to afford to build themselves, have sold or given free land to RSLs to develop in exchange for nomination agreements for lettings. These deals initially helped to keep down rents in new schemes, despite the high level of loan repayments on the debt. However, the level of private loans has increased as the proportion of development costs met by grants has been progressively cut, and this drove up rents significantly during the 1990s. The implications for RSL tenants are discussed in Chapter 4.

Since 1988 the sector has diversified and assumed a more commercial focus. RSLs have been involved in mortgage rescue deals with building societies, foyers for young people, Living Over The Shop schemes to bring back into use flats above shops, Housing Association Management Agreements to lease private dwellings to house homeless families temporarily and low-cost housing schemes in rural areas. They have been the main purchasers of council stock sold through voluntary transfers, and many are developing specialist supported housing schemes for vulnerable people under the care in the community programme. While improvement work to inner city housing has become more expensive and risky and has reduced substantially as a result, RSLs are moving away from building schemes on peripheral sites and working on smaller sites in inner cities as part of comprehensive urban renewal packages.

There are different types of RSL. Co-operatives provide housing to members only, who are more involved in the running of their homes than other tenants. Self-build housing associations use the members' own labour to provide the housing. During the 1980s the Housing Corporation developed a strategy to encourage black-led housing associations in order to cater more effectively for the needs of black people. This resulted in the creation of over 60 black and minority ethnic associations and co-operatives, although most are very small and need to work in partnership with larger (white) organizations to be viable.

Sharp cuts in grants in the mid-1990s brought a significant reduction in RSL development activity, intensifying pressure to merge or develop group structures to cope with the strictures of private funding. This reduced the role of the smaller, community-based organizations. RSLs found themselves in competition with each other for land and partnership deals with local authorities, and this threatened to erode the collective spirit of the movement. RSLs became increasingly dependent on borrowing private finance for development schemes and were constrained to charge high rents, which were not affordable by many households. Affordability is an issue of increasing importance for RSLs, with central government limiting rent increases as part of an overall strategy to keep downward pressure on Housing Benefit.

The changes described above relate to England and there are significant differences in the rest of the United Kingdom, as explained on pages 42–45. In 1989 the Housing Corporation's responsibility for Scotland and Wales ceased and its functions were taken over by Scottish Homes and Housing for Wales (Tai Cymru) respectively. In N. Ireland RSLs are directly controlled by the Department of the Environment, Transport and the Regions (DETR).

HOUSING FINANCE

Housing finance is a complex subject and this is not the place to present a comprehensive account of how it operates; others have done this effectively (see the Guide to Further Reading at the end of this chapter). However, an outline of the flows of money into and out of the housing system will set housing in the context of the national economic and social welfare policies, and will help to explain the massive tenure shifts which occurred during the twentieth century. Chapter 4 discusses the implications of this change for the cost of housing to consumers.

Housing subsidies

All government measures which affect the cost of housing can be called subsidies. Some reduce the cost of providing the housing; others reduce the cost to the consumer of the rent or mortgage. The major subsidies are listed by tenure in Table 2.1.

The total cost to the Exchequer of all the above subsidies did not fall in the 1980s and 1990s. However, there was a major shift in the balance of the subsidies, from underpinning the cost of providing housing towards underpinning the cost to consumers, i.e. from Column 1 to Column 2 in Table 2.1. Subsidies and grants to local authorities and housing associations were cut back, but the cost of Housing Benefit and MIRAS increased.

Table 2.1 Housing subsidies

Tenure	Subsidies which affect the cost of providing housing	Subsidies which affect the cost to the consumer
	Column 1	Column 2
Local authority	• subsidy to the Housing Revenue Account	• Housing Benefit
Registered Social Landlords	• grants from the Housing Corporation • loans from local authorities	• Housing Benefit
Private renting	• Business Expansion Scheme (now ended) • improvement grants from local authorities • Housing Investment Trusts	• Housing Benefit
Owner occupation	• improvement grants from local authorities	• Mortgage Interest Tax Relief (now ended) • exemption from capital gains tax • assistance with mortgage interest for those on Income Support • discounts on the price of homes bought under the right to buy

The government's definition of public expenditure is a very narrow one, covering the subsidies in Column 1 of Table 2.1. It is controlled by the DETR in England and N. Ireland and by the Welsh Office and the Scottish Office. This has been the focus of very severe cuts, directly affecting the activities of local authorities and RSLs. On the other hand, the main items in Column 2 are not defined as public expenditure on housing and do not come within the control of the DETR. Housing Benefit falls under the Department of Social Security, while MIRAS was regarded as tax foregone rather than money spent. It is these items which grew dramatically in the 1980s and 1990s, offsetting the cuts to public expenditure on housing.

The trends in expenditure shown in Figure 2.2 are best explained by examining each tenure in turn.

Local authority expenditure

Local authority housing finance in England and Wales is tightly controlled by the financial regime brought in under the 1989 Local Government and Housing Act. There is a clear separation between revenue and capital expenditure. On the revenue side, authorities keep a Housing Revenue Account which relates to the

Figure 2.2 Changing forms of assistance with housing costs for owner-occupiers and council and private tenants 1980/81–1997/98.

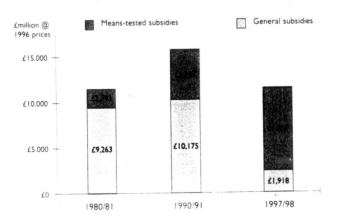

Source: Wilcox, S. (1998) *Housing Finance Review (1998/99)* York: Joseph Rowntree Foundation – Table 117b Assistance with housing costs for home owners, council and private tenants, £million at 1996 prices.

day-to-day running costs of the housing stock. On the expenditure side, the account covers the costs of managing and maintaining the council housing stock and the loan repayments on the debt raised for capital expenditure. The income side includes the rents received from tenants, Housing Benefit payments towards the rent for poorer tenants, and any DETR subsidy. This subsidy has been cut sharply since the early 1980s and very few authorities now receive any subsidy on their Housing Revenue Account. The era of the 'subsidized council tenant' ended some time ago. In fact, since the early 1980s the average amount of subsidy to each council tenant across the country has been less than the average value of MIRAS to each owner-occupier who has a mortgage.

'Surpluses' on Housing Revenue Accounts, which amounted to about £1.4 billion in 1998/99, have to be used towards the cost of Housing Benefit, and reduce the amount which the Department of Social Security has to pay in Housing Benefit for council tenants in that area. In effect those council tenants who pay the rent in full are contributing towards Housing Benefit for the poorer tenants. This system acts as a clear incentive to better-off tenants to leave the council sector and become owner-occupiers.

Local authority capital expenditure has to be kept under a separate account. This covers investment in the housing stock such as building new homes, major repairs of council housing, clearing land, loans to RSLs and improvement grants to owners. Capital expenditure is controlled through the annual Housing Investment Programme system, through which each local authority receives from DETR an annual 'credit approval', a maximum amount which it can borrow to finance the capital programme. In addition, authorities can spend up to 25% of the money received each year from selling council houses. In Scotland authorities have been allowed to spend all the money raised from sales until recently.

All such capital borrowing, together with the remaining subsidy to Housing Revenue Accounts, counts as public expenditure. This has been subject to the most severe cuts of any government programme since the early 1980s. While spending on law and order, social security, health and education has grown in real terms for most of this period, housing expenditure has been cut by more than half and is reflected in a virtual cessation of council new building and clearance, cutbacks in major maintenance programmes for council stock, and a significant fall in the number of improvement grants to private owners.

Registered Social Landlords

RSLs have also been affected by these cuts in local authority investment programmes, as loans to RSLs have been severely reduced. The main source of funding for RSLs is traditionally Housing Corporation grants and loans. Under the financial regime brought in by the 1988 Housing Act, RSLs now have to borrow privately to supplement the grants. This private borrowing is not counted as public expenditure, unlike corporation grants. In line with the policy of reducing public expenditure, the proportion of scheme costs met by grant was progressively cut from an average of 75% across all regions when the new system was introduced to just 54% by 1998/99. Intense competition for development approvals resulted in bids for developments with less than 40% grant support in some regions. The increasing reliance on private finance has driven both rents and Housing Benefit costs up steeply to cover the loan repayments.

Private landlords

The private rented sector has received little direct government support for providing homes. The major exceptions to this were the BES scheme and the support for Housing Investment Trusts, discussed on page 27. The introduction of Assured Tenancies and Assured Shorthold Tenancies in the 1988 Housing Act and the ending of rent controls for new tenancies has seen a sharp rise in rents in much of the private rented sector.

Rents have been driven up in all the rented sectors – local authorities, housing associations and private renting. This has been part of a broad policy to allow rents to reflect free market forces, while Housing Benefit takes the strain. The increasing cost of Housing Benefit reflects rises in rent levels and the increasing number of households dependent on benefits through un-employment and old age. The rise would have been even greater if local authorities were not increasingly contributing towards benefit payments for council tenants. There was also a series of cuts to benefit entitlements for many groups of households in the 1990s. Housing Benefit is now the single largest element of housing cost to the Exchequer.

Owner occupation

The other major growth in housing expenditure was MIRAS for owner-occupiers. MIRAS automatically reflected the state of the owner-occupied housing market. Its growth flowed from the

Table 2.2 Assistance with housing costs for individual households in Great Britain 1986/87–1997/98

£million at 1996 prices

	1986/87 (£million)	1990/91 (£million)	1997/98 (£million)
Owner occupiers			
Mortgage Interest Tax Relief	4,670	7,700	2,700
Means-tested assistance to meet mortgage costs	351	539	640[1]
Total	**5,021**	**8,239**	**3,340**
Local authority tenants			
General subsidies	1,356	1,468	(660)[2]
Means-tested assistance (Housing Benefit, rent rebates, Community Charge)	3,778	4,081	5,529
Total	**5,134**	**5,549**	**4,869**[3]
Private tenants			
General subsidies	–	127	–
Means-tested assistance (Housing Benefit, rent allowances, Community Charge)	1,167	1,573	3,790
Total	**1,167**	**1,700**	**3,790**
Total	**11,322**	**15,488**	**11,999**

Source: Wilcox, S. (1998) *Housing Finance Review (1998/99)*. York: Joseph Rowntree Foundation. Table 110 Housing Benefit Expenditure and Table 117b Assistance with housing costs and Table 101 Mortgage Interest Tax Relief

[1] Estimated out-turn
[2] This figure is a negative amount.
[3] Estimated out-turn: these figures are gross expenditure before deducting the contribution to their cost made by rent surpluses.

tenure policy of increasing home ownership, and was exacerbated by the house price boom of the late 1980s. A large number of economists advocated the ending of MIRAS, as it was costly, distorted the housing market and undermined a free market in prices. Various reductions were made from the late 1980s and MIRAS was finally abolished in the 1999 budget.

Other forms of support for home ownership are also significant, such as discounts earned by those exercising the right to buy their council home, and exemptions from capital gains tax on the sale of homes.

Table 2.2 shows clearly how the balance of the various housing subsidies for the three main tenures has been redistributed over an 11-year period. General subsidies to owner occupation through mortgage interest relief increased steadily until the early 1990s and then declined, while general subsidies to council housing disappeared and are indeed currently bringing a surplus into the Exchequer. Means-tested assistance, on the other hand, has increased in absolute terms in all sectors, especially for private tenants, despite several attempts by the government to rein in Housing Benefit expenditure and eligibility.

Building societies

As key financial agents for owner-occupiers, building societies have played an important role in housing finance. They currently provide over 60% of mortgage lending and have assets of over £300 billion. Building societies began in the eighteenth century as self-help savings and mortgage clubs, and members were predominantly the better-off working-class migrants to the expanding towns and cities. They have traditionally been mutual organizations, owned by the savers and borrowers. Their gradual expansion throughout the twentieth century is parallel to the growth of owner occupation (Stephens 1997).

Until the late 1970s, building societies dominated the mortgage market. They operated a cartel to fix mortgage interest rates, which kept rates below the market level and often led to excess demand and mortgage queues. They were cautious in their lending practices, particularly in refusing to lend in run-down inner city areas – a practice known as 'red lining'. In 1980, as part of a general policy of financial 'deregulation', other institutions including banks were freed from restrictions on lending for house purchase. Building societies' share of mortgage lending fell from four-fifths to about half during the 1980s. Societies also foresaw the levelling off in the future growth of owner occupation and sought to diversify their activities.

Building societies were given further scope to diversify under the 1986 Building Societies Act. For the first time, they could buy land, act as developers, set up estate agencies and develop insurance broking, share dealing and fund and unit trust management. They have also been able to develop a wider range of financial services including current account banking, personal loans and credit cards, insurance, pensions, Personal Equity Plans (PEPs) and Individual Savings Accounts (ISAs).

The relaxation of the rules restricting building society activity in 1986 had wider repercussions. They were allowed for the first time to raise money from institutional investors as well as individuals, and this led to a greatly increased supply of mortgage credit which facilitated the house price boom of the late 1980s. The 1986 Act also allowed societies to make loans for non-housing items secured on the value of property; where a house is worth more than the outstanding debt, the mortgage can be increased and the money spent on other things – a process known as 'equity withdrawal'. This helped to fuel the consumer boom of the late 1980s.

The 1986 Act also allowed building societies to convert to public limited company status, which could change them into banking institutions. The Abbey National was the first to convert in 1990 and many of the bigger societies such as the Halifax have since followed, marking a radical departure from their traditional role. Fierce competition, combined with the depressed housing market of the early 1990s, raised management costs and reduced efficiency. This has created pressure for acquisition and merger, causing branch closures and rationalization. From over 2,000 societies at the beginning of the twentieth century, the number dropped to 270 by 1980 and to fewer than 100 by 1998.

COMPARISONS WITHIN THE UK

Housing legislation normally applies to England and Wales, while Scotland and N. Ireland have developed separate frameworks. However, housing practice in Wales is not identical to England. This section will therefore look in detail at each.

Wales

The detail of interpreting the legislation is in the hands of the Welsh agencies: the Welsh Office under the Secretary of State for Wales, and Housing for Wales (Tai Cymru). Housing for Wales was established in 1989 to take over the role of the Housing Corporation in overseeing the housing association programme, and has developed its own approach. Wales has a higher level of home ownership than the rest of the UK and over a third of the property was built before 1919, compared with just over a quarter in the UK as a whole. Housing for Wales has recently developed a new regeneration programme to tackle areas of poor housing. There is also an acute lack of affordable homes in rural Wales and particular pressures from the second-home market. Under the Welsh Assembly a new department has been created, combining the functions of Housing for Wales with the housing division of the Welsh Office.

Scotland

Scotland also has its own Secretary of State and a Minister for Housing. The Scottish Office deals with local authorities, while Scottish Homes was set up in 1989 to oversee housing associations. As in Wales, Scottish local authorities have recently been reorganized into unitary authorities. Scotland has its own system of housing legislation, and while this largely mirrors policies in England and Wales, there are some important differences. Importantly, Scotland has had the same system of MIRAS and Housing Benefit.

The tenure pattern in Scotland has been very different from the rest of the UK with lower levels of home ownership and higher levels of council renting. The council stock particularly developed during the post-war slum clearance programmes in Edinburgh and Glasgow, much of it in high-rise flats on large estates. This prevalence of post-war high-rise housing, together with the traditional tenement form of building, means that a relatively high proportion of the population, over 40%, live in flats. Following the large-scale slum clearance activity there is a lower proportion of pre-1919 housing in Scotland than in the rest of the UK.

Since the 1980s there has been a significant shift in tenure, with declining council renting and rising home ownership, mainly through the right to buy for council tenants. Until recently Scottish councils were allowed to use all the capital receipts from these sales for new investment. As a result local authorities continued to build when building had virtually ceased in England and Wales. However, this freedom to spend all receipts has now ended; authorities were required to offset 25% of the receipts against debts in 1996/97 and this rose to 75% by 1997/98. There is a high burden of outstanding debt on the housing stock, which makes voluntary stock transfers less viable than in England.

When Scottish Homes was established in 1989 to oversee housing association activity, it also took over the stock of 75,000 dwellings from the Scottish Special Housing Association. It has embarked on a programme to dispose of this housing within the next few years, mainly to RSLs. The history of RSLs in Scotland is very different from that in England. There were very few RSLs prior to the mid-1970s, but there has been rapid expansion since, particularly of community-based associations and co-operatives with a major role in the rehabilitation of post-war housing estates.

Through most of the 1990s Scottish Homes also provided Grants for Rent and Ownership (GRO) to assist private developers to build or improve housing for sale and landlords to develop homes to let at market rents. These were focused on regeneration areas to bridge the gap between the cost of building and low values, and also in rural areas to reduce selling prices for priority purchasers.

The Scottish Parliament now has substantial authority over housing legislation and policy. However, its powers are constrained by the continuing influence of the UK Parliament over taxation and social security policy.

N. Ireland

The development of housing policies and structures in N. Ireland is unique. Throughout the first half of the twentieth century housing conditions declined and local authorities were not active in replacing the slums. Housing issues were predominant in the civil rights campaigns of the 1960s and housing authorities were accused of discrimination in the allocation of housing. The British government was forced to intervene and set up the Northern Ireland Housing Executive (NIHE) in 1971 to take over the functions of the local authorities. The NIHE is under the control of DETR N. Ireland and is run by an appointed board. It took over direct responsibility for a third of the total housing stock in the province and today has 140,000 dwellings, with both a strategic and landlord role.

Increased funding for housing in N. Ireland led to a major slum clearance and redevelopment programme in the 1970s, which continued on a smaller scale into the 1980s. This led to improvements in housing conditions overall. The record of the NIHE over allocations policy has been widely recognized as operating fairly. Around 20% of NIHE homes have been sold under the right to buy scheme. This has fuelled a rapid increase in owner occupation, which reached well over 60% by 1989.

There were very few RSLs in N. Ireland up to the mid-1970s and although the movement has grown since, it is still small compared with the rest of the UK. A new financial regime with mixed funding was introduced in 1992, several years later than in England. As in the rest of the UK, RSLs are increasingly expected to take on the public sector housing role, and now have the main responsibility for new building rather than the NIHE.

A review of housing in the province in 1996 suggested that responsibility for associations should transfer to the NIHE. This review also recommended that the NIHE should transfer its stock to housing associations and redefine its role as an enabler rather than a direct provider, similar to trends for British local authorities. The new N. Ireland Assembly has taken over the functions of all government departments including housing, but the NIHE has survived up to the time of writing.

KEY POINTS

- Today's housing stock is the legacy of the past; over a quarter was built before 1919 and under a quarter has been built since 1970.
- State intervention in housing towards the end of the nineteenth century was prompted more by political and social fears than by concern with the housing welfare of the poor.
- The First World War was a turning point in the history of housing policy, when it was recognized that the private housing market could not meet needs and the state had to play a key role in the provision of decent housing.
- There was a major shift in tenure during the twentieth century, with private renting falling from accommodating 90% of households to about 10% and a rise in owner occupation to approaching 70%.

- While the private sector was undergoing this transformation, local authority housing emerged to meet the needs of those not being catered for in the private market. Local authority housing peaked in 1979 and since then over one-and-a-half million homes have been sold.
- Housing associations have traditionally been small, independent agencies catering for specific groups of local people, but in the 1990s they have had an expanded role, taking on many of the functions of local authorities.
- The pattern of subsidies for housing has shifted away from support for providing housing through local authorities and RSLs, while support for consuming housing through rent and mortgage payments has risen.
- The system of housing finance is complex and anachronistic, favouring owner occupation above all other tenures, distorting the market and intensifying disincentives for many on benefit to find work.
- Building societies, many of which have become banks, are still the biggest source of funding for home ownership, but as the growth in home ownership slows down they have diversified into wider financial activities.
- Housing policy and practice differs in England, N. Ireland, Scotland and Wales, although the overall financial framework is similar in fundamental terms.

GUIDE TO FURTHER READING

Aughton, H. and Malpass, P. (1994) *Housing Finance: A basic guide.* London: Shelter.

This provides an admirably clear account of the complex regulations, subsidies and allowances in each of the main housing tenures. A valuable starting point, though inevitably slightly out of date.

Goodwin, J. and Grant, C. (eds) (1997) *Built to Last: Reflections on British housing policy.* Second edition. London: *Roof* Magazine.

A summary of articles which have appeared over the years in *Roof* magazine, providing accessible summaries of key points in the development of housing policy.

Housing as bricks and mortar

Outline

This chapter looks at the technical side of housing, from the perspectives of building, maintenance, planning and the environment. There is a huge backlog of repair in the public and private sectors with one in six dwellings in the UK needing urgent repairs costing more than £1,000. It has been recognized that tackling areas of poor housing requires physical upgrading and a wider package of improvements in design and management, and in the social and economic environment. Recent debates about where new homes should be built focus attention on the relationship between housing and planning, and the ability of the construction industry to cope with future demands. Housing design could cater better for the future by focusing on homes capable of meeting changing household needs and housing which is more energy efficient and environmentally sensitive.

HOUSING QUALITY AND CONDITIONS

Housing quality is a relative concept and is therefore difficult to define. Housing which was regarded as being of good quality a century ago is seen as poor quality today. Perceptions of the quality of a home are affected not only by its physical attributes but also by other factors such as a sense of security, the degree of control and privacy in the home, convenience of location, the neighbours and general feelings about the area (see pages 89–90). The actual experience of living in a dwelling is also determined by the number of people who live there and their income, which affects whether or not they can afford the rent or mortgage, keep adequate levels of heating and maintenance and so on.

Despite the difficulties in measuring quality, it can be argued that there are broad standards, which define acceptable housing quality in any one culture at any one time. These standards form part of the concept of 'fitness' defined in the 1989 Local Government and Housing Act, which applies to England, Wales and N. Ireland. Since 1969 a slightly different definition of fitness has been adopted in Scotland, the 'tolerable standard'.

The current definition of fitness is based on a list of physical factors, including both the presence of certain amenities and the state of the property.

The fitness standard

- piped water supply
- wash basin with hot and cold water, a fixed bath or shower, and an internal WC
- drainage and sanitation facilities
- facilities for cooking and food preparation, including a sink with hot and cold water and waste disposal facilities
- adequate natural and satisfactory artificial light, heating and ventilation
- substantially free from rising damp, penetrating damp and condensation
- structurally stable and in adequate repair

While some elements of the fitness standard can be technically defined, others remain a matter of opinion (e.g. 'adequate' and 'satisfactory'). The determination of 'unfitness' is a matter of skilled judgement rather than measurement. It is important to bear in mind that some key aspects of housing quality are not included in this fitness standard (e.g. adequate insulation, satisfactory layout of rooms and circulation spaces). The government is currently considering a major review of the fitness standard. Rather than being a checklist of items, the new standard may be based on a rating of the severity of each factor and its likely impact on the health and safety of occupants.

Since the 1960s there have been regular national house condition surveys. These surveys measure 'fitness', the presence of basic amenities (a kitchen, sink, bath or shower in a bathroom, wash basin, hot and cold water to each of these, an inside WC) and disrepair, measured by the cost of bringing the dwelling up to a specified standard. Comparisons over time are difficult because the definition of unfitness has changed and the interpretation varies within and between surveys. However, it is possible to gain a picture of housing conditions and trends in the UK in the mid-1990s.

- 1.7 million dwellings (7% of total stock) were unfit or below tolerable standard.
- Wales had the highest proportion of unfit homes – 13%.
- Disrepair is widespread, with one in six dwellings needing urgent repairs costing more than £1,000.
- One in five homes in England and three in ten in Scotland suffer problems of dampness, condensation or mould growth.
- Poor housing conditions are concentrated in the north of England, N. Ireland and rural Wales and Scotland, together with some London boroughs.

As Figure 3.1 shows, there appears to have been only a slight improvement in housing conditions during the 1990s.

Figure 3.1 Percentage of unfit dwellings in England 1986–1996

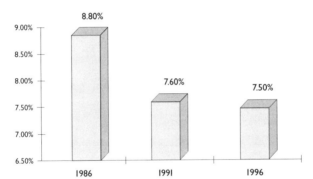

Source: Wilcox, S. (1998) *Housing Finance Review* (1998/99). York: Joseph Rowntree Foundation. Table 23b

There has, however, been significant improvement in the provision of amenities. In the early 1950s, over a third of dwellings had no fixed bath, and over one in twenty lacked an internal WC, piped water or kitchen sink. By 1991 virtually all households had access to a bath or shower, although over 100,000 households in Britain still lacked an internal WC.

There is a close relationship between the age of housing, its condition and the provision of amenities. The oldest housing tends to be in the worst condition. Terraced houses and converted flats are more likely to be in poor condition than other dwellings. Empty housing is most commonly in the worst state while the private rented sector has the highest proportion of stock in bad condition, with Houses in Multiple Occupation (HMOs) being particularly poor (see p. 53). The majority of homes in poor condition are owner occupied, because of the size of this sector. However, the scale of disrepair in council homes in England has risen during the 1990s.

Those who live in poor condition homes are most likely to be on a low income, to be older people or young people or ethnic minority households. Two-and-a-half million households of older people have no central heating. Of all households living in poor conditions in England in 1986:

- 13% were aged over 85
- 30% were low-income tenants
- 26% were low-income homeowners.

(Leather and Morrison 1997)

DEALING WITH PRIVATE DWELLINGS IN POOR CONDITION

This section focuses on:

- owner occupation
- grants for home improvements
- private rented dwellings.

Owner occupation

Although some owner-occupiers spend large amounts on repairing, upgrading and decorating their homes, the level of spending relates to income, with poorer homeowners spending least. Much of the work that is done is superficial do-it-yourself, to upgrade the appearance, such as decorations and kitchen fittings rather than basic repairs to the structure of the house.

Without state encouragement and assistance, many owners of poor condition housing would not maintain or improve the structure of their property for a number of reasons.

- Often the money spent does not raise the market value of the property by an equivalent amount (the 'valuation gap').
- It may be hard to raise a loan for improvement work.
- The home may not be perceived as unsatisfactory.
- There may be a distrust of builders or disinclination to face the disruption of building works.

If owners fail to keep property in good condition, this has wider implications. A legacy of poor housing for future generations builds up, the NHS has to treat illness resulting from unhealthy homes, and residential or community care services are needed where the home is unsuitable or unsatisfactory.

As discussion on the history of housing intervention (see pp.17–19) shows, the state long ago accepted a role in dealing with poor housing conditions. Clearance has been the traditional tool for dealing with unfit houses. However, the post-war clearance programme peaked in the early 1970s and 80% of local authorities have done virtually no clearance since the late 1980s. At the current rate of clearance, houses built today will have to last for 3,500 years before they are replaced.

Grants for home improvement

As the focus shifted from clearance towards improvement work, grants to owners to improve, repair and adapt their homes have been promoted. The grant system underwent a major revision under the 1989 Local Government and Housing Act and further amendment under the 1996 Housing Grants, Construction and Regeneration Act. The number of grants peaked in 1973–1974 and again in 1983–1984, in response to increases in the grant rates. Since the mid-1980s, the number of grants has steadily declined, the rate of decline increasing since the 1996 amendments.

Grants prior to 1989 were largely discretionary and there was great variation in local authority activity. They were not targeted on the worst condition properties nor given to lowest income households. A new means test for applicants was introduced in 1989 to target payments towards those most in need. In most cases, subject to the means test, grants were mandatory for unfit properties. However, this put an obligation on authorities which they found hard to meet, and in some areas informal waiting lists for grants developed. Under this pressure there was a disincentive for authorities to seek out and declare properties unfit, and the scope for discretion in the definition of unfitness was shown by the large variation in the number of grants paid in different areas. A limit on the amount of grant aid was introduced in 1993. It soon became clear that the system was unrealistic and it was amended in the 1996 Housing Grants etc. Act. The system is now once again mainly discretionary and comprises five main grants.

Home improvement grants

- A Renovation Grant can be used to bring a property up to the fitness standard, subject to a means test, the level of grant varying from nothing to 100% of the works required.
- A Disabled Facilities Grant may be given for adaptations and other work to enable a disabled person to live in their home, subject to a means test, with mandatory grants for certain work.
- A Home Repairs Grant may be given to help with insulation and replacement of lead pipes to people on benefit, older people and the disabled.
- A discretionary HMO Grant may be given to make the property fit and suitable for the number of occupants.
- A discretionary Common Parts Grant may be given to bring the common parts of a building containing flats up to the fitness standard.

In spite of the existence of grants, many owners are deterred from maintenance and improvement work by poverty, frailty and a fear of the upheaval of the works. Concern about the low uptake of grants by older people, the disabled and low-income households led to the introduction of Home Improvement Agencies in 1987 to provide practical help with repairs, improvements and adaptations. The funding of works can come from a variety of diverse sources including the five housing grants discussed above, social services, housing associations, charities and bank and building society mortgages. In the late 1990s the government provided additional funding for nearly 200 agencies in the UK. These are also supported by local authorities, housing associations (notably Anchor Housing Trust) and charities, and play a key co-ordinating role, often working with a range of agencies to enable a person to continue living in their home.

These agencies have been very successful in helping householders to negotiate the complex maze of systems involved in getting essential work done and paid for. Without this assistance, many older people would be unable to remain in their own homes, and would require residential accommodation, thus undermining the idea of care in the community.

The expansion of home ownership means that there are increasing numbers of low-income and older homeowners.

Allowing their housing to deteriorate would lead to long-term costs for society as a whole, such as increased health and social services expenditure and the need for demolition and clearance. With wholesale clearance being financially and politically unacceptable, it is important to provide effective incentives to owners to keep their property in good repair. These could include:

- continued and increased availability of grants
- further expansion of housing improvement agencies
- more imaginative loan packages for those who have the asset of a home but little income
- reducing VAT to 5% on repairs and renovation
- home logbooks to record work done and running costs
- sellers becoming responsible for structural surveys including estimates of maintenance costs (as would valuations)
- savings schemes for repairs including mortgages with a sinking fund
- improving public awareness of the need for maintenance.

In the late 1970s and 1980s, housing associations were also active in renovation, especially in the rehabilitation of run-down inner city areas and improvement area activity. However, the financial system for associations introduced in the 1988 Housing Act, combined with lower levels of grant and the requirement that associations bear the full burden of any cost over-runs, has deterred them and this work has virtually ceased.

Private rented dwellings

The private rented sector has the greatest proportion of poor housing. Local authorities have a range of powers to enforce repair and renewal of private rented housing under housing, environmental and public health legislation. These include powers to carry out works in default, prosecute owners, close the dwelling or demolish it. These are enforced by local authority housing and environmental health officers, often working together. Within the private rented sector HMOs are often in the very worst condition. An HMO is a house occupied by more than one household, and includes bedsits, shared houses and hostels. About two million people live in private HMOs. The law in relation to HMOs is complex with a plethora of provisions and regulations, most of them discretionary. Local authorities have powers to require physical improvements, provide grants to make properties fit, set standards of management and maintenance, limit the number of occupants, close the property, acquire it or take control of it. They are also able to set up an HMO registration scheme, and the government is considering a national licensing scheme for HMOs. A balance has to be struck between enforcing higher standards and retaining a stock of relatively cheap accommodation.

AREA IMPROVEMENT PROGRAMMES

Since the 1960s local authorities have been able to declare special areas where housing renewal activities are focused. General Improvement Areas (GIAs) were introduced in 1969 and Housing Action Areas (HAAs) in 1974. These were small areas covering a few hundred properties with a high incidence of disrepair.

The success of renewal in these areas depended on the willingness of owners to take grants and pay for the balance of the costs themselves. Often properties in the worst condition were owned by the poorest householders, who were unable to take part. Where the declaration of an area had the effect of raising the values of properties within it, this encouraged landlords to sell into owner occupation. This process was known as 'gentrification' and some areas experienced a high turnover of residents, with the original poorer households moving out and new middle-income owners benefiting from the improvement programme.

Often contrasts developed between the houses which had been improved and those which had not, and this undermined the concept of area improvement. As a result, 'enveloping' was introduced in 1978; local authorities could improve the external fabric of a block or street of private houses by repairing roofs, windows and walls. Enveloping was replaced by Group Repairs Schemes under the 1989 Act, with similar aims and slightly relaxed criteria. However, there has been limited uptake of these schemes, largely because grants are means tested.

The 1989 Act also replaced GIAs and HAAs with Renewal Areas. These are much larger, with between 600 and several thousand dwellings, but may also include commercial property and other land uses. The rules are that 75% of the houses must be unfit or in poor repair, 75% in private ownership and at least 30% of the households on benefits. Renewal Areas are more broadly concerned with urban renewal than were their predecessors, and a range of activities can be considered, including improvement, new building and clearance where appropriate.

By 1995, over 100 Renewal Areas had been declared in England and Wales. Like their predecessors, they have had limited success. This is partly because of the various restrictions on the type of area that can be declared a Renewal Area, which may exclude the worst parts of the inner cities. However, the main limitation is the continued fall in local authority resources.

SOCIAL HOUSING CONDITIONS AND URBAN REGENERATION

The huge cuts in local authority capital budgets in the 1980s and 1990s have affected not only support for private sector improvement but also the maintenance and improvement of councils' own property. House condition surveys show a deterioration in council stock during the 1990s, and the repairs and modernization backlog is estimated to be about £20 billion. Houses built before the war need modern amenities and heating systems, the post-war stock needs basic repairs, while many of the one million dwellings built in the 1960s and 1970s, using industrialized or system-building methods, have substantial problems of disrepair, including dampness.

In the 1980s local authorities were able partially to offset cuts in capital budgets by using money raised from council house sales, but as sales programmes slowed, this source of funding dried up. Those authorities with stock in the poorest condition tended to have the lowest level of capital receipts from sales because fewer tenants wanted to buy. The release of unspent capital receipts in the late 1990s has allowed an increase in renovation work but it has not compensated for the long-term fall in investment.

Many council dwellings in poor condition are on large peripheral estates, and it is now recognized that physical improvements need to be combined with a broader package of measures adopting a multi-agency approach, including:

- work specifically aimed at tackling security, such as changes to estate layout, stronger doors and locks, entry-phone systems, better lighting and landscaping
- management initiatives including a localized and intensive service, greater tenant involvement, receptionists or concierges in blocks, speeding up the reletting of empty properties, evicting

anti-social tenants, special lettings policies such as not giving flats in tower blocks to families with young children or setting aside particular blocks for certain tenants such as older people

■ social measures including the provision of play and social facilities and closer liaison with the police

■ local economic development such as training, education and employment development schemes, childcare facilities and using local labour.

These ideas have recently been taken up by RSLs in their 'housing plus' approach to development (see pp. 133–135).

The gradual recognition that housing upgrading has to be linked with social and economic improvements has been reflected in the various government schemes to tackle deprived areas, which are described below. The earlier programmes were primarily focused on housing improvements. Poverty among residents proved a major limitation on their success. More recent programmes have been part of wider regeneration packages with a greater focus on employment, training, transport and childcare. For more details, see Oatley (1998).

Government regeneration programmes

Many programmes were introduced in the last quarter of the twentieth century to tackle the very worst pockets of urban deprivation.

The **Priority Estates Project** (1979) used Department of the Environment (DOE) funds on selected estates to integrate estate-based management with the active involvement of tenants. These twin concepts of decentralization and participation have since been more widely adopted as part of housing management (see p. 135).

In **Estate Action** (1985) local authorities were required to bid for investment approval to tackle physical, management and social issues and establish estate-based forms of management with greater tenant input, or new forms of management such as tenant co-ops or management trusts. Partial sales of estates were encouraged to produce a greater tenure mix. Estate Action took an increasing share of total council housing investment up to the early 1990s, when it accounted for 20% of all local authority capital expenditure. The programme, involving over 1,000 schemes and 450,000 homes, brought significant improvements to some estates but was expensive, especially because of increasing management costs. By 1998 Estate Action was winding down.

Through the development of **Housing Action Trusts** (HATs, 1988), estates were to be transferred to a government-appointed boards with funding for improvement works. The government originally designated six estates but had to withdraw in the face of fierce tenant resistance. A HAT was eventually declared in Hull after the council gained significant concessions, including agreement that after completion the tenants could transfer back to the council. A small number of other HATs followed but the programme proved very expensive and was not extended.

City Challenge (1991) was based on partnerships between the public, private and voluntary sectors and linked housing improvements to industrial and commercial developments. Over 30 schemes were established. By 1998 the programme was winding down.

The **Single Regeneration Budget** (SRB, 1993) amalgamated a large number of different programmes across government departments, including HATs, Estate Action and City Challenge. It provides a comprehensive approach to the regeneration of the most deprived areas of public or private housing with partnerships between public, private, voluntary and community interests. The programme encompasses the economic, social and physical environment of an area with particular emphasis on jobs and education and lesser focus on improving housing, community safety and the local environment. The amount of money available for housing improvements within the SRB programme is considerably less than under the budget for Estate Action.

The **Estates Renewal Challenge Fund** (ERCF, 1995) had the more specific objective of extending the transfer of local authority housing out of the public sector. The fund was a dowry for the transfer of poor quality estates with a valuation that was negative or too low to attract private funding. This generally involved transfer to a new Local Housing Company or a new or existing housing association, together with a programme of improvement work (see p. 32). A small number of local authority bids were given DETR approval each year. ERCF was replaced by the New Deal for Communities.

The **Social Exclusion Unit** (1997) sets out yet another approach to areas of deprivation and has identified the worst 1,300 council estates. The unit aims to improve co-ordination between the various agencies working on the estates and to improve management. It concentrates on social rather than physical regeneration, and eighteen action teams have been established to promote policies to foster stronger communities and promote self-help. The action teams will focus on a number of key themes including neighbourhood and housing management, unpopular housing, anti-social behaviour and community self-help.

The **New Deal for Communities** (1998) is designed to target the most deprived neighbourhoods and includes measures to improve employability, to tackle welfare dependency and to provide support for an initial seventeen 'pathfinder' projects in neighbourhoods of about 2,000 homes. More areas will be able to bid for funds each year to provide resources to develop and implement local community-based plans covering everything from jobs and crime to health and housing. Residents must be the driving force in the programme of community regeneration.

Although the intention of these various programmes was to tackle the very worst pockets of urban deprivation, there is evidence that they have not been particularly successful. There is also concern that the focus on council housing misses out some of the most disadvantaged communities such as areas of low-income owner occupation in inner cities, often with a high proportion of ethnic minority households. While some estates have been improved, in other areas successive programmes have had limited success and decline has continued with rising unemployment and high levels of benefit dependency. The focus of improvement programmes has gradually widened out from mere physical upgrading to tackling more fundamental problems of social and economic deprivation, but it has yet to be demonstrated that any attempts at regeneration, however broadly based, can counter the powerful effects of poverty.

LAND AND PLANNING

Housing development has to compete against other land uses. The planning system plays a key role in the development of housing and helps resolve conflicting demands. The amount and location of land that the planning system makes available affects its price; land costs can be 40% of the price of a new house in high pressure areas. The planning system also affects the density of development, what sort of homes are built, the local environment and the long-term environmental impact of development.

Over the last two centuries the expansion of population and cities has brought a conflict between growth and the quality of the environment. The improvement in transport systems between the wars allowed development to spread over much larger areas than had previously been possible. The identification of a 'greenbelt' of protected land around cities, together with the designation of new towns, was devised to constrain this growth and prevent the continuous spread of urban areas.

However, the pressure continues. While the population of the UK is relatively stable, the number of houses required is growing as a result of higher levels of divorce and separation and an increasing number of single-person households. Government projections indicate there will be an increase of at least 4.4 million new households between 1991 and 2016 (DOE 1995). There is currently much heated debate about where the new homes for these households should be built. The pressure is greatest in southern England, especially in the shire counties and small towns and villages, but planning authorities here are fiercely resisting government targets for new building.

Options for new development include extending the boundaries of existing urban areas, developing new urban villages, and filling in unused land in urban areas. The government has set a target of 60% of new development being on urban spaces, known as 'brownfield sites'. These include abandoned industrial areas, land held by institutions such as hospitals and schools, open spaces and cleared land.

Many sites present difficulties. Development costs may be high due to the awkward shape of the site, or to the need to remove derelict buildings or foundations or deal with contamination from previous uses. Land prices may be high, reflecting the possibility of more lucrative commercial uses. The sale price of houses in inner cities may not reflect these high development costs, with the exception of certain popular schemes in particularly desirable locations. Although about half of new housing development has been on infill sites in the last few years, there is concern that this cannot be sustained, let alone raised.

Until recently, planning has been concerned with the number of new homes rather than their tenure and price range. However, pressure on the supply of land increases its price, which tends to lead to developments of more expensive homes and a lack of provision of new affordable housing. Even an increase in the supply of land may lead to only a small reduction in house prices because developers respond by building to lower densities. This problem was recognized in the early 1990s when the government's planning guidance adopted a new consideration for meeting a range of housing needs. Schemes above a certain size must now include affordable housing.

THE BUILDING INDUSTRY

The building industry is dependent on government macro-economic policy and has been badly affected by the downturn in investment in recent decades. Employment in construction accounts for about 7% of the total workforce, but the housing slump of the late 1980s and early 1990s resulted in high levels of unemployment. In the early 1990s there were well over half a million unemployed building workers and several major construction companies decided to pull out of the housing market.

The nature of employment in the building industry has changed as the industry has been fragmented and deregulated. It is increasingly dominated by a small number of giant firms, known as 'volume builders'. Their major activity is to develop land banks. Construction itself is subcontracted to smaller firms employing casual labour for each specific contract.

In contrast to house building, the house repair and maintenance industry is heavily dominated by small firms, employing seven or fewer employees. They are technically backward and often lack business skills. Techniques are labour intensive and innovation is discouraged. This may impede the development of new ideas for sustainable housing which respond to the needs of the future, as discussed on pages 63–65.

HOUSING STANDARDS AND DESIGN

Housing standards and design must take into account the characteristics of the people who will be living in the houses once they are built – including factors such as their income and their requirements for safety, comfort and accessibility.

Design for social housing

There is a direct relationship between the standard of housing and its cost, and hence the income bracket of household catered for. The growth of local authority housing between the wars was intended to improve living conditions and the 1918 Tudor Walters Report recommended what were then regarded as high standards for space, heating and facilities. These standards resulted in relatively high rents and restricted access to council housing to skilled manual workers who could afford the rent. It was also costly for the government in terms of subsidy. Council housing standards were gradually lowered during the 1920s and 1930s, both to reduce Exchequer costs and to bring rent levels within the reach of the slum dwellers being rehoused at that time.

After the war, when council housing was again built for general needs, space standards were raised in line with the 1944 Dudley Report, which applied throughout the building programme of the 1950s. However, the most comprehensive review of standards was the 1961 Parker Morris Report. This recommended minimum standards for floor-space in relation to the expected number of occupants, together with space for storage, household machinery, quiet activities and privacy; there was also provision for electrical installations and heating. These became the mandatory minimum standards for all local authority new homes from 1969. The need to meet these standards coupled with financial restrictions resulted in economies in materials which contributed to subsequent maintenance problems.

Parker Morris standards were abandoned at the end of the 1970s. Under increasing financial pressures, both local authority and housing association standards have declined, especially in terms of space. There is now concern that the decline in standards is building up problems for the future and creating a legacy of inadequate, unpopular estates which will be expensive to maintain. In an attempt to tackle the problem, the Housing Corporation issued new design guidance in the early 1990s but this is not mandatory and many associations are not adhering to it.

Before the Second World War, the design of council housing reflected the garden city model with low-density cottages. After the war the new design principles of the modern movement were adopted. This made use of technical innovations such as system building to create tower blocks. The new form of design was heavily promoted by large national building contractors, which gained substantial government support for industrialized building techniques. From 1956 to 1967 about half of all new local authority housing comprised system-built, high-rise flats and maisonettes.

Council housing at this time reflected the ideas of architects, planners and housing managers, with virtually no concern for what residents might prefer. As these estates gradually became unpopular, with emerging social problems such as crime and vandalism, some argued that their design features were directly affecting behaviour. The concept of 'defensible space' suggested a correlation between overlooked space – or lack of personally controlled space – and the incidence of crime and vandalism, and design alterations to estates were promoted as the solution. However, others argued against such physical determinism and saw estate problems as the product of far more complex and fundamental social and economic forces. While attention often focuses on high-rise estates, it is important to remember that until the early 1980s fewer than 30% of council dwellings were flats.

Private house building is subject to building regulations and planning controls, but has never been subject to minimum design standards, although the Parker Morris Report recommended that its standards should apply to the private sector. Rising land prices in the 1980s and the increasing demand for ownership from young, first-time buyers led to significantly lower space standards at the lower end of the market. Over half the private sector homes built in the early 1990s were below the Parker Morris space standards. This may be short-sighted: small homes are inflexible in their use and do not cater for future trends such as increased home-working, more home gadgets, more non-working households and greater leisure activities.

A reduction in overcrowding was a central aim of the early housing reforms, particularly to reduce the risk of infectious diseases, and there has been a steady decline in overcrowding since the 1920s. In 1991 fewer than 3% of households were overcrowded. Overcrowding particularly affects Asian households in older, owner-occupied houses, and lone-parent families in the social housing sector. Current standards for overcrowding date back to the 1930s and include two concepts: the space standard relates the sizes of rooms to the number of people living there; the bedroom standard ensures that no more than two people share a bedroom, nor do children over the age of 10 years have to share with children of the opposite gender.

Design for living

There has recently been interest in designing for those with limited mobility. One in four households will have a disabled member at some time and there are about 4.2 million severely disabled people in the UK. The increasing number of frail older people and emphasis on remaining at home have greatly increased the need for appropriate housing. Standards for homes suitable for people in wheelchairs and those with mobility difficulties were first introduced in the early 1970s, and councils and housing associations have for many years built a small number of specially designed homes, but currently only 2% of social rented homes are built to these standards.

Many other households would also benefit from more generous space standards, for example to manoeuvre baby buggies and accommodate visiting frail relatives. The concept of 'lifetime homes' has been developed to cater for the changing needs of households. Lifetime homes include accessible entrances, downstairs WCs accessible to wheelchairs, wider doors and circulation spaces and scope for a lift. Such homes cater for a variety of needs and lifestyles, and may enable people to stay at home rather than moving into residential accommodation. The idea has been pioneered in a few social housing schemes at an additional cost of a few hundred pounds; much less than the cost of adapting an existing house for a disabled person. There are similar arguments for incorporating lifetime homes features into rehabilitation schemes.

The idea of building to accessible standards will only have any significant impact if it also applies to private developments. There has been a long campaign to extend the Building Regulations Part M to ensure new homes are built to mobility standards. Private builders have been deeply resistant to any such requirements. However, the government has decided to extend these regulations to all residential development from 1999. The main cost is the extra space required, with greater costs for one- and two-bedroom homes but little effect on larger homes.

SUSTAINABLE HOUSING AND THE ENVIRONMENT

The issues discussed above are part of a wider debate about the kind of housing which should be developed in the future. This debate focuses on the concept of 'sustainable housing' which has a number of dimensions:

- house design, which should be flexible enough to cater for changing household needs

63

- locations which minimize the need for travel for employment and leisure facilities
- environmentally sensitive building materials, which should be renewable and not unhealthy or polluting
- energy efficiency including good insulation, provision for waste recycling and water conservation
- site location and density, which should use land with care (especially greenbelt and environmentally sensitive sites), minimize the need for infrastructure and reduce reliance on cars.

Recognition of the impact of site location and density on the environment has led to the concept of 'the compact city' for new land developments and attempts to increase the use of existing brownfield sites. Such new developments would be at fairly high densities to reduce the need for land, have mixed uses with employment and leisure facilities to reduce commuting and car travel, have good public transport, efficient waste recycling and the possibility of combined heat and power schemes (EDAW *et al.* 1997). This idea goes against the trend throughout the twentieth century towards dispersed cities and suburban development, but would be one way of balancing the conflict between the need for new homes and respect for the environment. This would require a new approach to land use and transport planning, and regional planning mechanisms and new incentives for the private water and energy companies to support savings in consumption.

The way housing is built, maintained and used has far-reaching implications for health and the environment. Homes which are cold or difficult to heat or have dampness, mould or condensation are unhealthy. Certain building materials such as asbestos and lead are known to cause illness; while others such as CFCs, tropical hardwoods which are not replaced and PVC which produces emissions during production add to global environmental damage. Landfill sites produce nearly half the UK's methane, which damages the ozone layer, yet little attention is paid to domestic waste recycling. Over a third of the water used is consumed in homes, with great potential for reduction.

Homes account for nearly a third of the UK's total energy consumption and produce over a quarter of all the carbon dioxide emissions into the atmosphere. Greater home energy efficiency could make a significant contribution to achieving the government's target of a 20% reduction in CO_2 emissions by 2010. While over four-fifths of dwellings in England have central heating, many of these systems are old and inefficient; it is estimated that a third of homes have unsatisfactory heating. Until recently, building regulations were not stringent in their requirements regarding energy efficiency and there was generally poor provision of insulation. As a result much of the housing stock has low energy efficiency. Many of these homes are occupied by poor older people who cannot afford the level of heating needed to achieve comfortable and healthy temperatures, and are in 'fuel poverty'.

There have been some recent attempts to improve energy efficiency. The 1995 Home Energy Conservation Act required local authorities to draw up plans for energy efficiency measures, although they received no additional budget to achieve this. The government's Home Energy Efficiency Scheme provides small grants for the provision of insulation and draughtproofing for low-income households of older people and Home Improvement Agencies assist older householders through the improvement grant system. Councils spend a significant proportion of their capital investment on heating systems and insulation, but this is from a falling budget. Several local authorities have pioneered innovative heating schemes to deliver affordable heating to tenants and the government has introduced a scheme for unemployed young people to install insulation as part of the Welfare to Work programme.

Sustainable development ultimately depends upon consumer support and community involvement. Consumers need better information about energy efficiency and construction quality when buying houses, and need to be convinced about the quality of life in more dense developments.

KEY POINTS

- About 1.6 million dwellings in the UK were classified as unfit in the early 1990s, while almost one in five dwellings in England needed urgent repairs costing over £1,000.
- Both slum clearance and private sector, grant-funded improvement work have greatly declined because of a lack of government funding. There are fears that the nation is storing up huge problems of poor housing conditions in the future.
- Local authorities are not adequately maintaining their housing and there is an estimated repairs backlog of £20 billion.

- There has been a number of different programmes for improving council estates focusing not only on physical upgrading but also on action to improve management and social provision, tackle crime and increase tenant involvement.
- Projections of the need for new homes to cater for the growth in households over the next few decades have led to heated debate about where the new homes should be built – on greenfield sites or unused land in the towns and cities.
- The construction industry is characterized by low investment, low productivity and high costs. Industry may not be able to respond to building demands in the future.
- Space standards have declined in both council and association new homes since the enforcement of minimum standards was abandoned at the end of the 1970s. Private homes are also being built to lower standards, and these small homes may not be flexible enough to cater for future needs.
- The shortage of homes suitable for people who have mobility problems has led to a call for the widespread adoption of 'lifetime homes' standards.
- Concern about what kind of housing should be developed in the future has generated the concept of 'sustainable housing', with flexible and energy-efficient design, and environmentally sensitive use of materials and land.

GUIDE TO FURTHER READING

For an up-to-date and detailed description of the condition of housing in the UK, see:

Leather, P. and Morrison, T. (1997) *The State of UK Housing: A factfile on dwelling conditions*. York: Joseph Rowntree Foundation.

For an interesting account of the relationship between housing and planning and designing for the future, see:

Goodchild, B. (1997) *Housing and the Urban Environment: A guide to housing design, renewal and urban planning*. Oxford: Blackwell Science.

For a comprehensive discussion of the impact of housing on the environment and the need for sustainable housing, see:

National Housing Forum (1997) *Living Places: Sustainable homes, sustainable communities*. London: NHF.

Housing
as home

Outline

This chapter focuses on people's experience of housing as home – who lives in what kind of housing, how they use and benefit from it and whether their homes meet their needs. It draws upon perspectives of sociology, social policy, economics and demography. An analysis of who lives where highlights differences between the housing of various types of household and demonstrates the increasing polarization between tenures, neighbourhoods and areas. Homelessness, the most extreme form of housing deprivation, is examined in a historical and policy context.

The perception of housing and preferences are partly determined by considerations such as availability, quality and cost. Status, ideology, and the sense of autonomy and control play key roles in housing choices. The meaning of home to the resident is influenced by the home itself and by the neighbourhood. Concerns about the increasing homogeneity of many housing estates have led to debate about social balance and attempts to engineer the social profile of local authority and housing association estates.

Finally the chapter shows that housing has a direct impact on educational opportunities, access to jobs and the likelihood of being a victim of crime. The concept of housing as home embraces the physical structure and the wider constraints and opportunities it confers; and the status, security, control and autonomy it provides.

HOUSING NEEDS

Housing needs depend upon the number, size and type of households. An increase in the number of low-income households, in particular, will create a need for more social rented accommodation. Each of these factors will be considered in turn.

Demographic trends

The number, size and type of households determine the need for homes. While the rate of population growth in the UK is slowing down, the number of households is increasing. Average household size has been reducing, largely due to the rising proportion of single-person households. This results from increasing numbers of older people living alone and a significant rise in divorce and separation. The growth in households of older people is predominantly among those over 75 years old. By 2025 it has been estimated that over a fifth of the population will be over 65 years old and they are likely to outnumber those under 15.

About 30% of households have children. As the number of married couples declines, the number of cohabiting couples and lone-parent families is rising. The majority of lone parents have been divorced, separated or widowed and under a third are single women. The image of large numbers of very young single women having babies is not borne out by the figures and lone-parent families tend to have fewer children than two-parent families.

Although there is some variation between ethnic minority groups, the broad demographic pattern is of a smaller proportion of older people but more family households.

Hidden households

People are only counted as households when they achieve a certain independent status. There is much greater need for housing than indicated by simple household projections. Many households live with another because they cannot get a home of their own; these include lone parents, couples and single people. Estimates of housing need have to make assumptions about what proportion of these 'concealed households' wish to live separately and should be catered for. Some will be able to obtain housing while others will be tomorrow's homeless.

Meeting needs

It is projected that there will be an increase of 4.4 million households in England between 1991 and 2016 (DOE 1995). This has implications for the number of new homes needed and also the type of homes which should be provided. There has been a heated debate about the balance between building new homes in inner cities and on greenfield sites, including arguments about sustainability (see pp. 63–65). Taking into account the fact that these households may not have sufficient income to become home owners, estimates suggest a need for an additional 90–100,000 social rented homes a year in the first two decades of the twenty-first century to meet household growth. To deal with the existing backlog of unmet need would require even more new social rented homes a year. However, fewer than 40,000 a year are currently being provided by local authorities and housing associations. This suggests that we are building up a serious housing shortfall in the next few decades, particularly for those who cannot buy.

These national calculations conceal significant regional variations. Regions with the slowest recent rate of growth are likely to continue to grow slowly, including the north-east, north-west, Yorkshire and Humberside, while the growth regions will continue to grow, including the south-east outside London, the south-west and especially East Anglia. This is reflected in significant regional variations in house prices and rents and in the demand for social rented housing. Homelessness is highest in the south-east, especially in London. In sharp contrast, in parts of the north of England there is such low demand for social rented housing that councils and housing associations have difficulty in letting properties, even those in reasonable condition.

WHO LIVES WHERE

This section looks at which types of household live in which types of tenure, and particularly the link between income and choice.

Household types and tenure

Table 4.1 shows which types of household live in which tenure.

Owners

Among owners, married and cohabiting couples predominate, while the high proportion of single female owners is made up largely of older women. In fact, over half of older people are now owners. This has implications for the upkeep of housing as they tend to have limited incomes for repairs, and for future levels of inheritance. The proportion of young single people who are owners in England is high compared with other countries, but there is evidence that this is changing. As job security reduces, the risks of ownership become more apparent, so fewer young people are leaving home before 25 and more are in further education.

Table 4.1 Percentage of tenure type by head of household

Head of household	Owner/ occupiers %	Social rented %	Private rented %
Men: Married	81	14	5
Cohabiting	63	22	15
Single	48	24	28
Widowed	63	32	5
Divorced/separated	50	36	13
Women: Married/cohabiting	74	16	11
Single	37	40	23
Widowed	56	39	6
Divorced/separated	48	40	12

Source: Wilcox, S. (1998) Housing Finance Review (1998/99). York: Joseph Rowntree Foundation. p118, table 29b. Note that all figures relate to 1996, save those for married and cohabiting women, which relate to 1995 as 1996 figures were unavailable.

Tenants of social housing

The majority of council and housing association tenants are families but with a much higher proportion of lone parents than among owners. Over half all lone-parent families live in the social rented sector. Households of older people form the other main group of social renting tenants. The existing social housing population is ageing while those entering the sector are young. The new tenants are increasingly likely to be unemployed and the profile of the sector is changing. The implications of this in 'residualizing' the sector are discussed on pages 72–74.

Private sector tenants

The private rented market caters for three main types of people: older people with long-standing tenancies, young mobile households including students for whom private renting may be a temporary phase prior to ownership, and low-income households unable to gain access to other tenures. Nearly one in five lettings is not generally available to new tenants because it is tied to a job or let to friends or relatives of the landlord. The expansion of private renting in the last few years has largely catered for young working households who are waiting longer before buying their own home. Private landlords are increasingly reluctant to let to those on Housing Benefit because of successive cuts and delays and uncertainties in administration, yet these households are the largest group seeking to rent privately.

Women and ethnic minority households

Black and ethnic minority households and households headed by women are disadvantaged in a variety of ways.

Women

Over 30% of households are headed by a woman. This generally means that there is no male adult in the household. Fewer than half all single, divorced and separated women are homeowners compared with over half such males and over three-quarters of married couples. This reflects the weak economic position of women-headed households; fewer women than men have full-time jobs and women's average earnings are lower than men's. Lone parents are predominantly female, are more dependent on social renting than other households, and are over-represented among homeless families and those in temporary accommodation. An increasing proportion of single homeless people are women, particularly very young women. However, women's homelessness is often hidden because they will put up with appalling domestic conditions including violence and abuse. At the other end of the age spectrum, the majority of pensioners are women, especially those over 75 years old.

Ethnic minorities

Black and ethnic minority households are similarly disadvantaged and tend to have limited housing options and live in worse housing than the white population. This reflects lower average incomes, but there is also evidence of discrimination in all sectors. This can take the form of direct discrimination where a black household is deliberately treated unfairly, or indirect discrimination where black people fall into groups which the system as a whole does not favour. Harassment and intimidation and the knowledge that certain areas or estates are unsafe also limit the housing options of black households.

When immigrant groups came to Britain in the 1950s and 1960s, they did not qualify for council housing as most councils excluded or gave low priority to those who had not been resident for a number of years. A high proportion of Asian households bought their homes, but could only afford poor quality housing in the inner city and had to depend upon high-cost loans from non-traditional sources because the building societies were reluctant to lend. This was reinforced by estate agents who directed ethnic minority buyers to certain areas. Many other immigrants turned to private renting but were confined to the poorer end of the market and had to contend with 'no coloured' signs.

Since the 1976 Race Relations Act there may be less overt discrimination but subtle discrimination remains. While many Asian owners still live in very poor condition homes in the poorest sections of the inner city, West Indian and African households have increasingly had access to council and housing association accommodation. However, studies have shown that they tend to be given the oldest housing stock with the poorest amenities, and a disproportionate share of flats rather than houses.

Residualization

A number of forces both within housing and arising from wider economic and social processes have resulted in the residualization of the social housing sector. This term refers to the increasingly high proportion of tenants who are disadvantaged, unemployed and dependent on benefits.

Until the 1950s council tenants were drawn from the better-off manual occupations with only a small proportion retired or otherwise not in paid work. The average income of council tenants was generally about the average for all tenures. However, from that time an increase in the number of older people as council tenants and increased numbers rehoused from slum clearance programmes resulted in a rising proportion on low incomes and not in work. The adoption of a national rent rebate scheme in 1972 assisted this process by allowing the very poorest to afford council rents. Councils have continued to focus on housing those in most need and from the early 1970s have housed increasing numbers of homeless households. This has been reinforced by the financial advantages of home ownership for those who can afford it, which has led to a shift of the better-off tenants out of renting into ownership, boosted by the right to buy programme from 1980 and more recently encouraged by rising rent levels.

The council sector has increasingly catered for a narrower range of types of people, as shown by measures of economic activity, wage levels, benefit dependency and the proportion of older people and lone-parent households. These groups are marginalized from the mainstream economy. There has been a significant increase in the proportion of the general population living below the poverty line as a result of changes in the nature of the job market, with permanently higher levels of un-employment, fewer unskilled manual jobs, more casualization and increased use of short-term contracts.

Housing associations are also experiencing residualization. An increasing proportion of new lettings is to those nominated by local authorities, including homeless households, and financial pressures have led them to build larger estates to lower standards. There is some concern that these estates will rapidly deteriorate and become unpopular or even unlettable in the future.

A higher proportion of new tenants are on state benefits, in receipt of Housing Benefit and unemployed, so the process of residualization is continuing. This is facilitated by the increasing rate of movement in and out of social renting, largely due to deaths among the high proportion of older tenants and partly as those who have jobs move out into owner occupation.

The residualization of the social rented sector is part of a wider process of polarization. Tenure differences are increasingly aligned with the distribution of wealth, resources and life chances. The social and spatial divide between owners and tenants has intensified, reinforced by deterioration in the type and quality of council stock as a result of right to buy sales of the better quality housing, the lack of new building and shortfalls in maintenance and modernization programmes.

However, the pattern of social deprivation does not coincide neatly with tenure. Within the social rented sector there is still a range of types of tenant and property, but there is a widening gulf between the more and the less desirable parts of the stock. The allocation process acts as a filter, as those in the most need will accept any accommodation while those in less urgent need will wait for a better offer. This is often formalized, for example, by giving only one offer of property to homeless households and refusing transfers to those in rent arrears. There may also be indirect discrimination against black and ethnic minority households (see

p. 130). Within the owner-occupied sector there is a growing gap between those who have benefited from price booms and those struggling to maintain their position. The continuing high rate of mortgage arrears and repossessions is evidence of this. A significant section of the owner-occupied market is low-value housing in poor condition, generally occupied by older people or Asians.

The residualization of social rented housing goes hand in hand with a range of other economic and social disadvantages. The new government concern with 'social exclusion' focuses on deprived council estates. Those with the least resources are trapped in an environment which provides the least support and fewest opportunities to overcome their disadvantage. Recent regeneration programmes have recognized this by combining property refurbishment with economic and social regeneration (see pp. 55–58). The new concept of 'housing plus' promoted by the Housing Corporation also couples housing development with broader economic and social projects (see pp. 133–135). However, it must also be remembered that social exclusion is not confined to council estates and in some places is more prevalent in poor-quality private renting or owner-occupied housing.

Rural housing

Rural areas are becoming increasingly polarized between the indigenous rural population dependent on insecure seasonal work paying low wages, and richer newcomers including people retiring to the country, commuters and owners of second homes. Demand for homes from new residents and the holiday industry pushes up prices and many rural areas have little housing which is affordable to local people. The cost of building also tends to be high because of transport costs, the shortage of land with planning permission and the need to build using expensive materials to conform to local styles.

Levels of rented housing, both public and private, are lower than in urban areas and there is a low turnover, accentuated by the right to buy, which has significantly reduced the amount of council housing in many rural areas. These pressures have increased migration of indigenous, particularly young, people from rural areas. This, coupled with the immigration of retiring households, has resulted in an ageing population. In response to the lack of affordable housing in rural areas, a planning 'exceptions policy' allows low-cost or social housing to be built in the greenbelt where need is demonstrable. However, this has not been widely implemented, partly because of high land costs.

Housing problems in rural areas tend to be less visible than in urban areas. Growing homelessness is often concealed by seasonal use of holiday accommodation or caravans as well as the emigration of those who cannot find anywhere to live. Old country houses may look attractive but the percentage of dwellings in poor condition is higher in rural areas than in urban ones.

HOMELESSNESS

This section considers those who have no secure housing of their own. The impact of homelessness on people's lives, particularly their health and welfare, is discussed in Chapter 5.

Homeless people

Homelessness can be seen as a continuum ranging from roofless people to those in inadequate or insecure housing.

The homeless continuum

- without a roof
- in homeless accommodation: e.g. shelter, hostel
- in insecure housing: e.g. bed and breakfast, holiday let, squatting, short-life housing
- shortly to be released from an institution: e.g. care, hospital, prison
- sharing accommodation where relationships are intolerable: e.g. violence, abuse, family breakdown
- living in unsatisfactory accommodation: e.g. unfit, too small, wrong location, too expensive
- sharing involuntarily

Homelessness affects families and single people and is the product of a wide range of factors – housing, economic and social. The amount of housing available and its cost underlies trends in homelessness, with a recent reduction in both public and private renting and higher rents and house prices, especially in the regions of growth. This has been coupled with economic constraints and with higher unemployment, benefit cuts and widening geographical inequalities in job opportunities. At the same time, long-term social trends – with higher divorce and separation rates, rising numbers of older people and the growing desire of the young to live independently – have increased the need for housing. Taking these factors together, it is not surprising that homelessness rose in the 1980s and 1990s. The greatest incidence occurs in areas where there is a shortage of rented housing and of houses to buy at the lower end of the market, and where a high proportion of the population is dependent on benefits. However, while in general homelessness is greatest in London and the south-east, it has been rising faster in other areas and is a problem in rural as well as urban areas.

The homeless are not a homogeneous group. Young people may leave home with little support and be unable to get a foot on the housing ladder. Some may become homeless at the point of forming a household and starting a family, while families may become homeless at a point of crisis such as job loss or separation. Some people spend much of their life in institutions – the armed forces, hospital, prison – and never find secure housing in between. Some homeless people have many problems and need support and care as well as housing, while others simply need somewhere secure to live at a price they can afford.

The state's response to homelessness

The state has taken long-term responsibility for helping certain homeless people, distinguishing between the 'deserving' and the 'undeserving'. Under the Poor Law, workhouses catered for homeless people from the district and there were punitive regimes. The Poor Law was replaced by the 1948 National Assistance Act, which required county authorities to provide temporary accommodation for people in urgent need. Until the late 1960s homeless people were categorized as disturbed, and homelessness was attributed to personal inadequacy. It was treated as a welfare issue and housing authorities were not generally involved. The county authorities' duties applied predominantly to families with children, although they were often split up with fathers excluded from the hostels or children taken from their parents and put into care. The National Assistance Board provided Reception Centres for single homeless people.

During the 1950s and 1960s there was mounting pressure to see homelessness as a housing issue, reflecting housing shortages rather than individual failings. The TV play *Cathy Come Home* and the launch of Shelter added impetus to this pressure. In 1974 a government circular recommended that housing authorities take over homelessness duties from social services departments (DOE/Department of Health/Welsh Office Circular 18/74). However, most local authorities did not implement the recommendations. After protracted debate it was finally accepted that the circular needed legal enforcement, culminating in the passing of the 1977 Housing (Homeless Persons) Act.

The 1977 Act placed a duty on housing authorities to secure accommodation for people in priority need and to advise and assist others. The priority groups included families with children or a pregnant woman, and single people vulnerable through age or mental or physical disability. The interpretation of the Act was detailed in successive Codes of Guidance. The legislation was always controversial, some seeing it as a charter for the feckless and others seeing it as too limited in its scope. By denying rights to those with no local connection and those who had rendered themselves 'intentionally homeless', it retained the distinction between the deserving and undeserving, and by focusing on families it gave few rights to single people.

These provisions, consolidated in the Housing Act 1985 and the Housing (Scotland) Act 1987 and extended to N. Ireland in 1988, stood for nearly two decades until replaced by the Housing Act 1996. This followed several reviews of the legislation, prompted by lobbying by those who saw the homeless as queue jumpers and scroungers, and in the context of increasing pressure on local authority lettings. The 1996 Act follows the format of previous legislation with a number of 'hurdles' which a homeless applicant has to surmount before the housing duties come into play.

The homelessness hurdles

- Eligibility – primarily a question of immigration status – those from abroad are generally excluded.
- Homelessness – defined quite a way along the continuum (p. 75) to include domestic violence and accommodation which it is not reasonable to continue to occupy.
- Priority need – priority need groups are: pregnant women, those with children, the vulnerable, and those who have lost their home because of a natural disaster.

- Intentionality – those who have lost their home through their own fault are excluded from assistance.
- Local connection – in some circumstances applicants can be referred to another area.

Once an authority is satisfied that an applicant is eligible, homeless, in priority need and not intentionally homeless, the rehousing duty comes into play. The major change of the 1996 Act was to make this a time-limited duty (two years), and also to limit access to permanent social housing, which could only come through a waiting list application (see p.121).

Households accepted by local authorities

Prior to the 1977 Act, local authorities already had to accept increasing numbers of homeless people. The numbers continued to grow throughout the 1980s and early 1990s, but have since declined, as is shown in Figure 4.1.

Figure 4.1 Acceptance of homeless households (England)

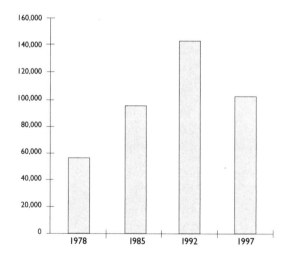

Source: DoE and DETR *Annual Homelessness Statistics.* London: HMSO.

Homelessness – the statistical picture

- Over 100,000 households were accepted by English local authorities in 1997, 4,297 in Wales and 16,800 in Scotland.
- These households include over a quarter of a million people, half of them children.
- The fall in acceptances in the 1990s has occurred in all areas.
- Over half of those who approach local authorities as homeless are turned away because they are not in one of the statutory priority need categories.
- Over a quarter of those accepted are sharing accommodation with family or friends who are no longer willing to accommodate them, often with only one room for the family.
- A further quarter have become homeless following relationship breakdown.
- A growing proportion of acceptances follows the loss of a private rented home, about 22% in 1998.
- The proportion of people becoming homeless after mortgage arrears rose to a peak of 12% in the early 1990s but has since declined.
- Homelessness often follows a sequence of events involving temporary housing situations that eventually break down.
- A high proportion of homeless households have never had a secure home of their own.
- Over half of those accepted are families with dependent children and a further 10% include a pregnant woman.
- There has been a steady increase in single people accepted because they are vulnerable in some way.
- Those accepted include a disproportionate number of ethnic minority households and a very high proportion are unemployed and dependent on benefits.

Responses in practice

There are wide variations in how local authorities interpret their duties. For example, authorities differ in whether they accept those discharged from long-stay psychiatric hospital, women without children experiencing domestic violence, those under 18 and those living in statutorily unfit accommodation.

The acceptance of homeless households rose during the 1980s when new building was falling and authorities were losing housing through sales. Homeless households took a growing proportion of lettings. This reached a peak in the early 1990s with just under 40% of all new council lettings being given to homeless households. In some parts of the country the pressure was even greater with nearly all homes suitable for families allocated to the homeless. Councils made more use of their nominations to housing associations, which grew to the point where nearly half of all new association lettings were to the homeless.

The increased numbers of homeless households reduced the rate of rehousing from ordinary waiting lists. This generated heated debate about queue jumping. Reviews of homelessness legislation in the early 1990s and the changes brought in by the 1996 Housing Act reflect this view of the homeless as less deserving. However, three-quarters of those accepted as homeless are already on the waiting list and do not constitute a different group, merely those whose need has reached a crisis point (Audit Commission 1989). If local authorities had been still building and letting on the scale of the 1960s and 1970s, these same families would have had a chance of rehousing from the normal waiting list before their situation became urgent.

Temporary accommodation

Housing authorities place homeless households in temporary accommodation for a number of reasons. In some cases they are waiting for the results of investigations into their circumstances prior to a decision being made, in others there is a shortage of suitable permanent housing, while in some areas it has been used as a deterrent to those whose need may be less urgent or less genuine. Overall about a third of those accepted are initially placed in temporary accommodation. This includes hostels, refuges, bed and breakfast hotels, short-life housing and properties leased from the private sector.

- The use of temporary accommodation increased throughout the 1980s to a peak of over 63,000 households in 1992.
- Since then, the increased supply of housing association property and the decline in acceptances enabled the figure to fall to about 44,000 by late 1997.
- Bed and breakfast hotels have been used extensively, with about 12,000 households staying in them at any one time in 1991, but the number had reduced to just over 4,000 households by late 1997.
- Authorities use about 9,000 places in hostels for the homeless, many of which they own.

Much temporary accommodation, especially bed and breakfast hotels, provides appalling conditions which have a detrimental effect on residents who may be there for considerable periods of time (see p. 96). Temporary accommodation is also very expensive, and in many areas homeless families have to be placed outside the local authority area because of a shortage of suitable local temporary accommodation.

Because of the high cost of bed and breakfast hotels and their poor quality, authorities have made more use of private sector leasing in the 1990s and it now forms the majority of temporary housing. There are various different arrangements, with some leased from the owner by authorities and managed either by the authority or a housing association, and some being leased by associations who take council homeless nominees. Although cheaper than bed and breakfast, rents tend to be high and may not be fully covered by Housing Benefit. The supply of temporary private sector housing is not secure and owners may withdraw their property to sell as the housing market picks up. Some authorities are also using up the local supply of private renting by permanently discharging their duties to the homeless through referrals to private rented homes. There are fears that the private sector may not have the capacity to meet the need for both temporary and permanent accommodation for the homeless, and authorities may have to make more use of bed and breakfast hotels in the future.

Homeless people not accepted by local authorities

Every working day nearly 1,000 households approach local authorities seeking help with homelessness. Well over half are not accepted because they fall outside the provisions of the legislation, including many vulnerable single people. In addition, many others do not even approach councils for assistance because they do not believe they qualify. Because local authorities do not have rehousing responsibilities towards those who are not accepted, there are no reliable figures on their numbers, but estimates suggest there may be over one-and-a-half million people, including a quarter of a million young people.

These 'hidden' homeless people are in a variety of circumstances and include those sleeping rough, squatting, staying in hostels, lodgings or insecure private lets, women living with violent partners, travellers and people living in caravans and boats, and people sharing with others who wish to live separately. They are not a homogeneous group and many move frequently from one insecure situation to another. Among those who use hostels and bed and breakfast hotels are increasing numbers of young people and a disproportionate number from ethnic minorities (Anderson, Kemp and Quilgars 1993). While most are men, there are increasing numbers of women, particularly very young women, living in hostels and hotels. The number of young people who sleep rough has also increased although the majority are older people. A high proportion of single homeless people have spent some time in an institution such as a children's home, hospital, prison or remand centre, with perhaps a quarter having been in the armed forces.

In spite of the Children Act 1989, which places a duty on social services departments to provide accommodation for young people in need, agencies dealing with young homeless people find that up to a third have been in care (Centrepoint Soho 1996). The number of those under 18 years old using winter shelters has risen steeply, with more girls than boys using them. Young homeless people have often experienced violence or abuse and have been particularly affected by the cuts in Housing Benefit for those under 25 and income support for those under 18 years old.

The scale of street homelessness increased visibly in the late 1980s, particularly in central London. In response, the DOE Rough Sleepers Initiative was launched in 1990. It initially provided money for emergency hostels and housing association temporary and permanent housing in inner London. The programme has since been extended to provide more permanent housing and to cover areas outside London. The success of *The Big Issue* has also raised the profile of the problems of the street homeless. The initiative has reduced the numbers of people sleeping rough and a new government approach in the late 1990s aimed to deal with those remaining. However, there remains a core of people sleeping rough whose problems are so complex that programmes to bring them off the streets have yet to meet with success.

Although local authorities have been able to reduce their use of bed and breakfast hotels (p. 80), many other homeless people rely on this as accommodation of last resort, especially in traditional seaside towns and urban centres. These single people and families who are not eligible for housing authority assistance include refugees and asylum seekers, care leavers and people with mental health problems. They lack security of tenure and are vulnerable to harassment and eviction. Social services departments also place people, mainly destitute asylum seekers, in hotels,

HOUSING COSTS AND BENEFITS

Housing not only reflects patterns of poverty but can exacerbate disadvantages for some while providing opportunities to others. This is underpinned by the distribution of personal housing costs and benefits. Chapter 2 discusses housing finance and government subsidies. This directly affects individual housing costs and the options and opportunities available to households.

Tenants

As a result of the withdrawal of housing subsidies to organizations (see p. 38), average weekly council and housing association rents in England have risen by more than 100% between 1988/89 and 1997/98. There are large regional differences reflecting development costs and market demand. New housing association rents are particularly high and in parts of the north of England they are on the same level as free-market private sector rents.

These rent rises have created problems of affordability. There is no agreed definition of what is an affordable rent, and the Tory government in the late 1980s simply referred to rents within the reach of those in lower-paid employment. Attempts to identify a guideline level have generally put rents at between 25% and 35% of net household income. The majority of new housing association lettings are above the National Housing Federation's guideline of 25% of net income. As a result those in work have a strong incentive to move out of the sector and only those on Housing Benefit can afford to move in, thus exacerbating the trend towards residualization (see pp. 72–74). About two-thirds of current social renting tenants are on Housing Benefit compared with about 85% of new housing association tenants.

The problem of rising rents has been recognized by the Labour government of the late 1990s and measures have been introduced to limit both local authority and housing association rent rises. These rents continue, however, to rise at above the rate of inflation.

Those who get Housing Benefit may not be directly affected by the level of rent but do face a 'poverty trap' if they look for work or extra earnings. They may lose Housing Benefit and other income-related benefits if they earn. Many households face a financial disincentive to seek work at the prevailing wage levels and many others lose substantial amounts of any wage increase by the loss of benefits, amounting to effective tax rates of 90% or more. The housing finance system traps tenants in unemployment and inhibits them from taking up opportunities.

The system of housing allowances, channelling assistance for rent through Housing Benefit, imposes a severe poverty trap. Cuts in Housing Benefit introduced in 1996 restricted 100% cover to rents at or below average for the area. Only 50% of rent above this level is covered by Housing Benefit, and the rest is not met by social security payments but must be found by the householder. A significant proportion of tenants are affected by this restriction.

Some former tenants, however, did very well, being able to take advantage of generous discounts through the right to buy.

Owners

Affordability has also become an issue in the owner-occupied sector. Lower-income groups have been encouraged into ownership through a combination of push and pull factors. Access to social rented housing has become more difficult in many parts of the country, while the poor condition of much of the stock, the lack of new building and sharply rising rents have made this option less attractive. On the other hand, there have been generous discounts under the right to buy scheme and the liberalization of the finance markets in the 1980s made it easier to borrow a higher proportion of both income and house value.

However, owners with maximum mortgages have been badly affected by the increasing insecurity in the labour market which has reduced both job security and take-home pay levels, and by progressive reductions in the value of MIRAS. In addition, the prevalence of variable rate mortgages linked to current interest rates makes the cost of repayments particularly volatile. Mortgage arrears and repossessions rose sharply in the early 1990s. In 1991 nearly a million owners owed two or more months' payments and repossessions were over 1,500 a week. Since then there has been a downward trend although the figures remain high. The reduction partly reflects the housing market recovery in the 1990s and partly more sensitive practices by lenders.

The Housing Benefit system has never applied to owners. Owners are assisted through the Income Support system, which covers mortgage interest payments. Since 1995 this has been available only after the first nine months out of work. In any case three-quarters of borrowers in arrears have no claim on the Income Support safety net. The most vulnerable owners tend not to take out insurance cover for loss of their job.

In sharp contrast to the difficulties of marginal owners, others have made large gains from the housing market. Inheritance is becoming increasingly important as a form of wealth accumulation and nearly two-thirds of all inherited wealth is in the form of property. Three-quarters of inherited property is sold immediately and nearly half the money is invested, while about a third is used for buying or improving a house and the rest used for general spending. The number of inherited properties is likely to double in the next 30–40 years and it is estimated that by 2025 there could be a million beneficiaries. However, if the number of older people selling their homes or extracting the equity to pay for residential care increases significantly, the value of inheritance will not rise as fast as projected.

Inheritance accentuates existing inequalities. It is disproportionately distributed to higher social classes, existing home-owners, and those in London and the south-east, while children of homeowners tend to marry other children of owners and thus stand to gain from two inheritances.

HOUSING AS HOME

British housing policy is much more dominated by tenure than is the case in other countries. Tenure preferences are shaped by considerations of finance, availability and quality and also by ideology. Home ownership has been promoted by Conservative governments and by Labour administrations. Indeed, the 1965 Labour government housing White Paper described the spread of home ownership as 'normal' and the 1977 Labour Housing Policy Review called it 'a basic and natural desire'.

This long-term support of home ownership was accentuated in the 1980s by Conservative governments often accused of having a tenure policy rather than a housing policy. Here, a desire to increase home ownership and reduce social renting was underpinned by a fundamental belief in the superiority of one tenure over the other. One Tory MP made this very clear: 'Council housing is only for those who, whether through poverty or lack of moral fibre, cannot make the grade as owner occupiers – a second class sector of second class people' (quoted in Griffiths 1982).

The meaning of home

Surveys have shown a rising preference for home ownership among non-owners. Some sociologists (notably Saunders 1990) have seen this as reflecting a natural desire to own. In this view, home ownership provides a sense of security, autonomy, privacy, belonging, personal identity, choice, expression, achievement and pride. But there is more to the experience of 'home' than tenure. Perceptions are shaped by memories of major life events such as forming of new relationships, children growing up and bereavement. The experience of home is affected too by the way in which the house is designed and used, relationships with neighbours and community, and the division of domestic labour in the household. What makes a house a home is a complex web of factors. The balance between them varies with age, race, class and gender. 'Home' has been summarized as:

> an index of social status, an arena of intimate relationships, a refuge, a container of possessions and icons, and even the carrier of one's self-image
>
> (Ravetz 1995)

The preference for owner occupation may have less to do with its ability to confer security and more with government policies (especially favourable tax treatment of owners) and the difficulties associated with other tenures, such as poor conditions, problems of access and perceptions of bureaucratic management. In addition, the preference for home ownership reflects a desire for a range of physical attributes including space, quality, a house with a garden and a particular location. These are not tenure specific but may be more easily obtained by buying than renting.

Neighbourhoods and social balance

One of the key influences shaping people's feelings about their home is their perception of their neighbourhood. Satisfaction surveys on council estates often reveal that people like the interior of their home but dislike the external environment. This has been accentuated by the process of residualization in the social rented sector, polarization between tenures and the increased spatial segregation of neighbourhoods.

The concentration of disadvantaged households is blamed for creating undesirable neighbourhoods, reinforcing social and management problems, creating a spiral of decline and under-mining stable communities. One response has been to promote 'social balance' on estates. The idea is not new and was adopted by the garden city movement before the First World War and by the new town programme after the Second World War. The council building programme after 1945 was intended to cater for a wide range of social groups and create mixed communities.

The recent renewed search for social balance has led to innovations in allocation policies and the promotion of 'community lettings schemes' in some neighbourhoods, which take account of factors other than acute housing need. Priority may be given to people with local ties or to adult children of existing tenants, while those with children of a certain age or households with a known history of anti-social behaviour may be excluded. Many such schemes also aim to give tenants greater involvement in the running of the estate. This approach has been applied to existing difficult-to-let estates and also to new estates to prevent similar problems developing. However, there is limited scope for social landlords to manipulate social balance and the long-term benefits of community lettings are unclear.

Another approach to achieving wider social balance and more stable communities is to introduce a mix of tenure on estates. There have been experiments with mixed and flexible tenure schemes, including a form of shared ownership which allows residents to switch between renting and owning as their circumstances change (Joseph Rowntree Foundation 1996).

However, social balance is not widely sought by tenants and most people prefer to have neighbours of a similar background to themselves. Tenants' main priorities are choice about where they live, good local facilities, effective management (especially to deal with neighbour conflicts and local crime) and more involvement in the running of the estate.

Most of the problems faced by social landlords stem from wider social and economic processes such as poverty, crime and unemployment. Rather than try to deviate from the basic principle of housing those in greatest need, it may be more effective to link housing development with programmes which aim to tackle these broader problems, such as the 'housing plus' initiatives as discussed on pages 133–135, and broader-based renewal programmes (see pp. 56–58)

Inequalities and opportunities: education, jobs and crime

Where you live affects your health and access to health care (see Chapter 5), education and job opportunities, and exposure to insecurity and crime, and confers a status or stigma which itself determines access to other services. In this way the housing system shapes and sustains inequalities. These disadvantages not only affect those who live in inadequate housing but also generate costs which fall on other services such as health, education, social services, the police and the criminal justice system, and have a wider impact on society and the economy.

Education

Housing can affect opportunities throughout life. It is harder for children in a poor home environment to achieve success at school. Overcrowding, a lack of quiet space for study, cold and damp, and increased illness can all hamper their ability to learn. The education of children in homeless families is particularly disrupted by their enforced mobility and inability to settle in one school. Young children in bed and breakfast hotels may have developmental, behavioural and psychological problems (Conway 1988). All this can create lifetime disadvantages. The special educational needs produced by poor housing also increase the demands on educational services.

Jobs

The cost and location of housing affects job opportunities. For many households the combination of high rents and the benefit system creates a disincentive to work, because most additional income from employment is lost from benefits, leaving them little better off (see pp. 83–84). The location of housing in relation to employment markets is also important. Work opportunities are reduced where the jobs involve long journeys, high fares and reliance on poor public transport services. Large peripheral housing estates often isolate residents from employment, reducing the opportunities and incentives for work. Frequently, these areas are also have poor childcare provision, again reducing employment prospects. Homeless people experience particular problems as their frequent need to change address can make a permanent job inaccessible.

There are large regional imbalances in housing which restrict labour mobility and may inhibit economic growth. The south and south-east have shortages of rented housing and high house prices, while in parts of the north social rented housing is difficult to let and prices are considerably lower. The regions with most employment opportunities are also areas of housing pressure. It is difficult to move from one region to another to obtain work. Employers in the south-east report a lack of suitable labour, while there are pockets of very high unemployment elsewhere. Investment in new housing construction is itself a potentially significant source of new job opportunities.

Crime

There is a heightened general concern with crime in Britain. However, crime creates particular anxieties on some social housing estates, which have become associated with vandalism and graffiti, burglary, assaults, drug distribution and abuse, car theft, noise and harassment. Council tenants are nearly twice as likely to be burgled as owner-occupiers. Crime also has wider effects on residents, including increased expenditure on security and insurance, a fear of crime – which restricts going out, especially at night – and dissatisfaction with their housing which can lead to stress and ill-health. Housing agencies have to spend more on repairs, anti-vandalism measures and security devices for flats and blocks, and lose rent because of the greater number of empty properties. The criminal justice system has to bear the cost of policing and prosecution. Agencies spend considerable amounts on dealing with the results of crime and on preventative measures to make homes safer and more secure. These form a key part of most estate renewal strategies (see p. 58).

The perceived level of crime and anti-social behaviour in an area plays a major role in determining its reputation. This affects the price and marketability of private houses and the popularity of rented houses. Areas can become stigmatized, with many consequences for residents' lives. Insurance policies and loans may become prohibitively expensive or impossible to obtain, local shops may close, GPs and school teachers may not be attracted to work in the area, buses may not run at night, and taxis may be reluctant to come to the address. It has even been suggested that having a particular address reduces employability.

To summarize, therefore, in many direct and indirect ways housing can affect people's health, education and job opportunities, vulnerability to crime and access to services. Poor housing can have a detrimental impact on those who are already disadvantaged and exacerbate inequalities. The costs of this fall on the residents and also on other services. Ultimately the whole society and economy has to bear the cost of poor housing.

KEY POINTS

- Demographic changes have increased the need for homes, especially for the growing proportion of single-person households. Estimates of future needs for social rented homes far exceed current levels of building, suggesting a growing shortage of housing for those who cannot buy, particularly in the south and south-east of England.
- Households headed by women are at a disadvantage in the housing market, reflecting their weak economic position. Similarly, black and ethnic minority households tend to live in worse housing than the white population, partly because of lower average incomes but also due to discrimination and harassment in all housing sectors.
- Long-term social, economic and housing forces have resulted in the residualization of the social housing sector, with increased concentrations of disadvantaged tenants in poor quality housing. There is a widening social and spatial divide within each housing tenure, between owners and tenants and between neighbourhoods.
- Rural areas are becoming increasingly polarized between richer newcomers who can afford the high housing costs and the indigenous population who are being priced out.
- The increase in homelessness stems from housing, economic and social factors and may be seen predominantly as either a housing or a welfare issue.
- Local authorities have a duty to assist certain homeless people and this has placed rising pressure on the shrinking stock and increased the use of temporary accommodation.
- The single homeless population includes growing numbers of young people and women, and a significant proportion have multiple problems requiring a range of support services.
- The distribution of personal housing costs and benefits exacerbates disadvantages for some while providing opportunities for others.
- What makes a house into a home is a complex web of factors including ideology, choice, security, personal identity and memories and the neighbourhood. Some see the rise in home ownership as reflecting a deep and natural desire to own while others see it as the product of long-term government housing policies which have favoured ownership above all other tenures.

- One approach to increased residualization has been to promote a greater social mix on social rented estates by altering allocation policies to take into account factors other than need. However, there is limited scope for social landlords to manipulate social balance on any significant scale.
- Housing segregation accentuates existing social and economic inequalities by placing the most disadvantaged people in locations which further reduce their life opportunities. Where you live affects your health, educational and job opportunities, exposure to insecurity and crime and access to a wide range of other services.

GUIDE TO FURTHER READING

For a rather dated, but still the most comprehensive view of the impact of gender and race on housing, see:

Morris, J. and Winn, M. (1990) *Housing and Social Inequality*. London: Hilary Shipman.

For a more detailed view on women and housing, see:

Gilroy, R. and Woods, R. (1994) *Housing Women*. London: Routledge.

For an interesting perspective on the meaning of home, particularly for owner-occupiers, see:

Forrest, R., Murie, A. and Williams, P. (1990) *Home Ownership: Differentiation and fragmentation*. London: Unwin Hyman.

For a detailed account of the homeless persons' legislation, its history and interpretation by the courts, see:

Arden, A. and Hunter, C. (1997) *Homelessness and Allocations*. Fifth edition. London: LAG.

Housing, health and social care

Outline
This chapter focuses on one major perspective on housing – health and social care. Following increasing inequalities in society there has been a concentration of vulnerable people into council and housing association accommodation. This has brought new demands on social landlords and highlighted the importance of housing to health and social care agencies.

THE RELATIONSHIP BETWEEN HOUSING POLICIES AND HEALTH

The emergence of housing policies in the nineteenth century arose directly out of a concern with health (see p. 18). The urban slums were centres of infectious disease, crime and poverty that threatened the health and stability of the cities. During the cholera epidemics, doctors saw at first hand the appalling conditions and were among those who spearheaded campaigns for public action. It can be argued that improvements in housing and the environment have had a far greater effect on the general health of the population than any advances in medicine.

Nineteenth-century reformers believed that state intervention in housing would break the link between poor housing and poor health. The removal of the worst slums in the nineteenth century, and again in the 1930s and 1950s, was assumed to deal with unhealthy housing once and for all. During the twentieth century the focus of housing policy gradually drifted away from dealing with poor quality housing towards other issues such as ownership and management, access and cost.

In the last decade or so there has been a renewed awareness of the fundamental relationship between housing and health among both housing and health professionals. From the housing perspective there has been a realization that bad housing conditions persist. Improvement activity in the private sector is failing to keep pace with deterioration. Some local authority blocks of flats are also in very poor condition, affected by severe dampness, condensation and unaffordable heating.

From the health perspective there has been a realization that health inequalities persist. A new recognition of poverty has undermined assumptions about the effectiveness of the welfare state. Bad housing exacerbates the health problems of the poor. They live in the worst housing, cannot afford to heat their homes adequately and experience water disconnections. Homelessness could be regarded as living in the most extreme form of unhealthy housing and there are shocking figures on morbidity and mortality rates among the homeless, as discussed on page 96. The care in the community policy has also brought into focus the essential links between housing and health (see p. 109).

This renewed recognition of the links between the environment and health is reflected in the government's public health strategy produced in the late 1990s. Health action zones which adopt a holistic approach to improving health and provide an opportunity for housing to play a part have been introduced. Health authorities have to produce health improvement programmes and all programmes must be assessed for their health impact. This broader approach to health recognizes the underlying causes of ill-health, including housing, and once again sees housing as contributing to the nation's health strategy.

THE EFFECTS OF HOUSING CONDITIONS ON HEALTH

There is a wealth of evidence to show that good housing is crucial to good health (Arblaster and Hawtin 1993). The relationship operates in two ways:

- Poor housing conditions can directly cause or exacerbate physical and psychological ill-health.
- Housing can create conditions which foster disease, e.g. causing stress which brings vulnerability to ill-health.

Damp, mould and condensation are linked to a range of illnesses including respiratory diseases, asthma and allergies. Cold homes can increase chest disease, heart disease and strokes and can result in hypothermia. Older people are particularly vulnerable yet live in the worst heated and insulated homes. Two-and-a-half million households of older people do not have central heating. They are among those who experience fuel poverty: inability to afford adequate warmth because of the home's energy inefficiency. Poor people tend to spend a higher proportion of the day at home than better-off households and are more affected by the conditions; they also spend a higher proportion of their income on heating despite living in colder homes.

There is a number of government programmes to improve heating and insulation (see pp. 63–64). The provision of better heating and insulation has been shown to improve residents' health and reduce demand on the health service. However, these programmes have not been carried out on a sufficient scale to prevent the apparent increase in fuel poverty.

Poor housing conditions underlie very many of the accidents in the home which result in about two million people needing hospital treatment each year, most of whom are older people and children. Over 4,000 of these accidents are fatal, making up about a third of all fatal accidents. Home accidents cost the NHS over £300 million a year, to which must be added the cost of lost working time. In addition there were over 800 deaths from house fires in 1996. Poor wiring is one of the main causes and risks are particularly great in Houses in Multiple Occupation (HMOs).

There is increasing understanding of the health effects of poor air quality and certain materials in homes. Radon gas can build up in homes and is the largest source of exposure to radiation for many people; it can cause lung cancer. Poorly installed and maintained heating installations can result in carbon monoxide poisoning. Building materials dangerous to health include lead (used for water pipes), asbestos, some types of foam insulation, and certain types of wood preservatives and pesticides.

The provision of basic facilities in homes has steadily improved. Good quality water, effective waste disposal and adequate facilities for food storage and preparation are essential to avoid bacterial infections. Well-maintained sewage systems are necessary to keep out rats but there is evidence of a recent explosion in the rat population. Overcrowding fell steadily in the twentieth century but still occurs, especially in the ethnic minority population. It has been linked to cardiovascular and respiratory diseases, accidents, depression, the spread of infectious diseases and slow development in children.

House type also affects health. System-built housing is particularly prone to cockroach infestation in the ducting. These spread germs and disease and may cause allergic symptoms and stress. Poor sound insulation may be linked to mental ill-health. Families with young children can be adversely affected by living in high-rise flats which lead to isolation and stress in mothers, and slow development and respiratory illness in children.

The neighbourhood can also affect the health of residents. People living in unpopular estates have been shown to experience isolation and insecurity and are more prone to respiratory diseases, stress and depression. Areas with a poor local environment (dirty, dimly lit, with a lot of traffic and other sources of noise, crime and vandalism, etc.) are also likely to lack health promoting facilities (parks, recreational facilities, local shops selling healthy food, etc.) and all this is often further compounded by poor local primary health services.

Studies have found it very difficult to establish a direct causal link between housing conditions and ill-health because of the presence of other factors such as poverty, overcrowding, poor diet and so on. However, anyone working with those who live in poor-quality housing is aware of the detrimental impact of those conditions on both their physical and mental health. There are also wider economic implications. The health service has to provide more GP consultations, prescriptions and hospital out-patient and in-patient services for housing-related conditions such as asthma, heart and respiratory problems, home accidents and stress-related illnesses. The Department of Health has estimated the cost to the NHS of illness from condensation in the home alone to be £800 million a year. Hospital discharge may be delayed where the home is unsuitable, resulting in bed blocking. Days lost through illness impede children's learning in school and are a drain on employers and the economy as a whole.

Government and local agencies are becoming increasingly aware of the links between housing and health and some are developing local schemes and strategies to tackle them together (Chartered Institute of Housing 1998). In some cases health authorities have supported housing improvements to reduce ill-health in poor quality homes. These innovations depend on effective joint working, discussed on page 110.

HOMELESSNESS, HEALTH AND SOCIAL CARE

The context of homelessness is discussed in Chapter 4, including underlying factors, the range and circumstances of people who become homeless and legal duties of local housing authorities. This section focuses on health and care needs of homeless people.

Health problems of homeless people

The link between homelessness and ill-health has a number of dimensions:

- Illness may lead to homelessness.
- Homelessness brings an increased risk to health and may exacerbate health problems.
- Homelessness is associated with unhealthy behaviour such as alcohol or substance abuse together with a high risk of violence.

People living on the streets and in temporary accommodation experience particularly severe health problems. These stem both from their poor living conditions and also from the stress of insecurity and enforced mobility. Examples of health problems suffered by homeless people and those living in temporary accommodation are given in Table 5.1.

Table 5.1 Health problems of homeless people

Families in temporary accommodation	Single homeless people
• poor diet	• chronic chest and breathing problems
• infections	• malnutrition and digestive problems
• child accidents	• infestation and skin complaints
• poor child development and behavioural problems	• musculo-skeletal and foot problems
• stress and depression	• dental, eyesight and hearing problems
• obstetric risk for pregnant women	• risk of violence and assault
• babies born with low birth weight	• mental ill-health

Families in bed and breakfast hotels live in cramped and overcrowded rooms with all their possessions. Toilets, bathrooms and kitchens (where they exist) are often unhygienic and shared with many other families. The lack of sound insulation is stressful. Poor maintenance increases the risk of accidents, especially for children who are confined to their room or play on staircases. Pregnant women are at risk and babies born to women living in hotels tend to have low birth weights (Conway 1988).

Single homeless people tend to move between hotels, hostels and sleeping rough. They experience a poor diet, insanitary conditions, vulnerability to cold and personal risks. The insecurity of homelessness is very stressful and leads to isolation, difficulties in getting medical care and schooling, and inability to get a job.

Single homeless people have a particularly high incidence of multiple physical and mental health problems. There is an increasing incidence of TB among homeless people and the average age of death of homeless people dealt with by the inner London coroner's court in 1991/92 was 47. Suicide is the biggest single cause of death among the street homeless. It is estimated that about a third of those sleeping rough and those in hostels and hotels have mental health problems compared with 5% of the general population. A significant proportion have been in-patients in a psychiatric hospital, yet are not receiving regular support under the care in the community policy. Disorders include schizophrenia, depression, self-harm and drug abuse.

Agencies have identified 'the revolving door syndrome' whereby people with complex problems fall between services and move round from the streets to hospital to prison and back to the streets again. There is a core of people in many inner cities who have been rejected by hostels and direct-access centres as too disruptive, yet are not regarded as ill enough to stay in hospital for more than short periods. A study of men remanded to Winchester prison for psychiatric reports over a 4-year period found that nearly two-thirds were homeless on arrest (quoted in Arblaster and Hawtin 1993). A third of these had been charged with burglary and theft including many minor incidents. Moreover, prison offers many mentally vulnerable people the care and treatment that they cannot get elsewhere.

Access to health care

Coupled with their health problems, homeless people have very poor access to health services. Homeless people have particular difficulties registering with a GP and may get only temporary registration, so their medical notes are not forwarded. This partly reflects their inherent mobility and tendency to delay seeking medical help until a condition is acute. There is also evidence that doctors are reluctant to treat homeless people, whom they perceive as more expensive to treat than the resident population. As a result, homeless people make greater use of hospital Accident and Emergency Departments than the general population and have a greater incidence of hospital admission. This is an expensive form of health provision.

The complex nature of the needs of single homeless people was recognized by the establishment of the Department of Health Homeless Mentally Ill Initiative at the beginning of the 1990s (in parallel with the DOE's Rough Sleepers Initiative) providing outreach community mental health teams together with hostels and move-on accommodation. In some areas local health agencies provide specialist services, including specialist GPs, outreach teams for street homeless people, mobile clinics and health care services in hotels, hostels and day centres. Some health authorities have dedicated nurses and health visitors for the homeless.

When homeless families and single people are re-housed, many continue to need support to maintain their tenancy. This cannot be provided by housing agencies alone but requires the co-operation of a range of services, as discussed on pages 110–111.

VULNERABLE PEOPLE

Some groups of people have particular needs which require special consideration. These include the homeless, disabled people and frail older people, people with mental health problems, those who are HIV+ or who have AIDS, young vulnerable people, travellers, refugees and asylum seekers. Having considered homeless people, this section focuses on three other groups. The numbers of disabled and frail older people are large and rising while the reduction in institutional provision means that more are living in the community. Similarly there are many people with mental health problems who need both decent housing and support. This requires housing agencies to work closely with care and health agencies. The number who end up homeless indicates the difficulties of achieving this. Their needs highlight the importance of good housing practice which all housing agencies should aim for in the interests of all households.

Disabled and frail older people

There is a strong overlap between these two groups. Many people become disabled late in life and over two-thirds of the disabled are older people. There are also many young disabled people who live with parents or in an institution and have few housing choices. The term 'disability' refers to a loss or limitation of opportunity owing to social, physical, or attitudinal barriers.

Over six million adults in Britain have a significant physical impairment and one in seven households includes someone with a disability. This includes four million adults with mobility difficulties, while 1–2% of adults use wheelchairs. Others have difficulties with hearing, sight and using their hands and the biggest single cause of impairment is arthritis. The number of people with a disability has been rising because there are more older people, particularly frail older people, and medical advances increase the numbers surviving accidents and disease. The care in the community policy has reduced the use of institutional care and further increased the need for suitable housing.

Disability has more to do with how society treats you than with personal characteristics. Someone with an impairment can be disabled by their environment and made dependent. For example, a person in a wheelchair who can move about easily on smooth floors at home will be disabled by steps at a day centre. Suitably designed or adapted housing is crucial both to facilitate independence and to minimize the costs of support services.

Most older people and disabled people do not live in institutions and do not wish to be in segregated special needs housing schemes. Over half the households of older people are now homeowners, but many cannot afford to keep their home in good repair or pay for adaptations as they become frailer. Their homes may prejudice their health and prevent them from remaining independent. Improvement Grants and Disabled Facilities Grants available from housing authorities help low-income households, while social services, health authorities and housing associations can assist with home adaptations. The most common adaptations are stair lifts, showers and wheelchair ramps. Demand for home adaptations has increased sharply in the 1990s, but funding for grants has been severely restricted. The process of achieving improvements and adaptations is complex, lengthy and uncoordinated and many are deterred from even applying. The average time from applying for an adaptation to completion is over a year; such delays result in additional costs to the state in terms of care.

New building also makes a contribution to the stock of housing suitable for frail older people and disabled people. Councils and housing associations have been designing a small proportion of their homes for those with mobility difficulties since the early 1970s. Much of this has been one-bedroomed housing, although many disabled people live with others. The fall in social rented new building in the 1980s and 1990s reduced this supply to a trickle. Many social landlords have a stock of sheltered housing for less frail older people; this is discussed on page 103.

More recently the idea of 'lifetime homes' has been pioneered in a few schemes, with enhanced access and circulation space to cater for a range of mobility needs (see p. 63).

People with mental ill-health

Mental illness is common. Depending on the definition used, between one in ten and one in four of the adult population are experiencing mental illness at any one time, while about 1% of the population is estimated to have a severe mental illness. There are now well over 100,000 fewer psychiatric hospital beds than 40 years ago. Alternative provision such as supported schemes has increased but most people with mental illness live, and prefer to live, in ordinary housing. People with mental health problems need accommodation which is appropriate, affordable and safe. Those on a low income will only be able to afford poor-quality private sector housing. Social landlords may recognize their needs through the medical priority system, being identified as homeless and vulnerable, or nomination by health or social care agencies. However, the accommodation which is immediately available is often the most unsuitable, in hard-to-let areas which may feel isolating, unsafe and threatening.

As well as decent accommodation, many people with mental health problems need some kind of support, which may range from companionship, housekeeping and financial advice, to medical and psychiatric support. The community care system tends to focus on the most acute needs and there is a shortage of low-level, preventative support. For some, particularly street homeless people, this lack of suitable housing and support makes it difficult or impossible to maintain a tenancy.

As well as the serious human cost, poor provision for people with mental health problems results in greater costs in other areas. Health and care services may have to rush in to provide intensive support to deal with a crisis. Tenancy failure is costly to a social landlord as it incurs rent loss, staff time to reallocate the property and often the cost of boarding up the premises or repairing deterioration and vandalism while it is empty. For the health service, a significant proportion of short-stay psychiatric beds are unnecessarily occupied by people ready to be discharged but who lack a suitable package of housing and support. Homeless, mentally ill, people often fall foul of the law and increase demands on the police, probation service, courts and prisons.

The link between housing and mental ill-health operates in a number of ways. Mental illness can result in housing problems. There is also evidence that housing problems and homelessness in particular can lead to or exacerbate mental ill-health, particularly anxiety and depression. The physical condition of a dwelling can also undermine mental health.

The closure of hospital beds and the care in the community policy have increased the numbers of social tenants with mental health problems. Many are not getting the care support they need and housing managers have to take on a more complex set of tasks, as discussed below. The needs of this group highlight the importance of agencies working closely together to provide a seamless service, not just for those recognized by the care in the community programme but for many other vulnerable people.

THE ROLE OF HOUSING AGENCIES

Increasing numbers of people have complex needs requiring some form of support and the current policy emphasis is on minimizing the use of hospitals and residential settings so that vulnerable people can live in the community. Most of those with the most acute needs are provided with a care package under the care in the community programme, but this is often dependent on them having a suitable home to live in. Many more have less severe problems and are not entitled to support from social services or the health service. They live in ordinary – often social rented – housing, and the housing service may be the only agency in regular contact with them. As a recent Audit Commission report summarized:

> Health services have refocused on acute care; social services have targeted their resources on higher-level needs and continuing care,

leaving housing providers to cope with chronic needs that require ongoing support

(Audit Commission 1998 p. 13)

Housing agencies carry out a wide range of functions dealing with health and social care needs which are summarized below:

- Provision of suitable housing
  - good quality housing
  - rehabilitation to improve energy efficiency
  - new housing for disabled tenants
  - adaptations to social housing
  - grants for adaptations and improvements to private homes
  - support for home improvement agencies
  - sheltered housing
  - hostels
  - supported housing
  - furnished accommodation

- Access to suitable housing
  - sensitive response to all applicants
  - advice and re-housing for homeless vulnerable people
  - medical priority applicants
  - involvement in community care assessments
  - matching disabled applicants to property
  - accepting people coming out of hospital, care, prison, etc.

- Housing management and support
  - day-to-day management support
  - housing advice
  - sheltered housing wardens
  - community alarms
  - specialist support staff
  - benefits advice/debt counselling
  - help with resettlement
  - liaison with other services and agencies
  - services for those in temporary accommodation
  - community work on estates

Provision of suitable housing

Most people require good quality ordinary housing in a safe environment with sensitive and responsive housing management. Social landlords provide a range of forms of housing for those with health and social care needs. However, following decades of cutbacks in social housing services, local authorities and housing associations are often only able to provide accommodation on unpopular poor quality estates which is not healthy, supportive or safe. It is ironic that the shift towards vulnerable people living in the community in ordinary housing rather than in institutions has occurred just at the time when the ability of the council housing sector to supply decent healthy housing has fallen. Many vulnerable people end up living in environments that undermine their ability to cope and in some cases this precipitates a crisis that then requires an expensive response from other services. There has been a concentration of vulnerable people into poor areas and this is a challenge to housing management, as discussed below.

Some people need a more specialized form of accommodation. In addition to facilitating specially designed or adapted housing for disabled people in both the public and private sector, housing agencies provide sheltered housing, hostels and a range of supported schemes. Local agencies ought to measure needs in their area and plan strategically to meet them. However, there is an acute lack of local information and provision tends to be the result of inherited uncoordinated decisions. There is little relationship between the supply of specialized housing and local needs.

Sheltered housing for older people is by far the most common form of specialist housing. There are nearly half a million sheltered dwellings with an on-site warden, similar to the total of residential and nursing care places. This comprises an average of 11% of council and 21% of association housing. These schemes usually provide self-contained dwellings in a block with communal facilities such as a common room and laundry room. Most are purpose built but a few have been created by converting other property such as tower blocks. In addition there are schemes for more independent older people with a visiting warden and no communal facilities, while some 'very sheltered schemes' provide intensive care support for those who are very frail.

While demand for very sheltered housing has risen, demand for traditional sheltered housing has been falling and most social landlords have some that is difficult to let. It may not be catering for current needs. In particular the role of wardens needs rethinking. They have traditionally played the part of 'good neighbour' but are increasingly called upon to deliver more intensive care and even medical assistance. Rules about the use of housing authority accounts limit the extent of care support which housing authority wardens can give, while restrictions on what Housing Benefit may cover also constrain the level of care supplied. Higher levels of care may be appropriate but can only be provided in collaboration with other agencies.

Community alarm systems are increasingly extended beyond those in sheltered housing schemes. These provide an emergency alarm or voice contact linking someone at home to a central station that sends immediate assistance. In many areas this is available to older people in private housing and can be used for other vulnerable people such as the disabled or those under threat of personal violence. It provides reassurance and support to those living independently. Over a million people are connected to a community alarm.

There are many types of hostels and supported accommodation. Hostel accommodation has a long history. Poor Law authorities provided workhouses for destitute families and ran basic shelters or 'spikes' for single homeless people. After the welfare state was introduced council welfare departments provided hostels for homeless families; these are now largely run by housing authorities. The National Assistance Board took over the large short-stay reception centres for single homeless people. The Department of Health and Social Security later ran these as resettlement units but they have now largely been replaced by smaller hostels run by local authorities and voluntary organizations. Other agencies also provide hostels, particularly the Salvation Army which has about 50 catering for up to 5,000 homeless people. Housing associations have also developed a range of smaller hostels, often for specific groups of people such as those with learning difficulties or young homeless people.

While hostels are largely seen as offering temporary refuge prior to more permanent settlement elsewhere, some people prefer to be in a hostel than in their own flat because it can offer companionship, security and a high level of support. In addition, some hostels are designed to give more permanent accommodation. Many residents have health and care needs. However, most hostels lack the resources to care for those needing very high levels of care or with behavioural, drug or alcohol problems. There is also a shortage of hostels for women and those with disabilities and of hostels where black people feel at ease. Foyers are a recent innovation providing accommodation and support with training and job access (see p. 132).

Other forms of supported housing schemes often cater for those with more severe health and care needs. Provision expanded significantly in the 1980s and is now diverse, including blocks of special-needs accommodation, group homes and 'core and cluster' schemes where a core of services is provided to people living in different forms of dispersed housing. Some schemes are for permanent residents while others are designed for short-term support prior to moving into independent accommodation. They play a key role in the care in the community policy and form part of a web of local provision, sometimes linked to day centres, peripatetic support services and more intensive accommodation. Housing associations are major players, using Supported Housing Management Grants from the Housing Corporation to fund the higher levels of management (not care or support) required. Management is often a partnership arrangement with a combination of housing association, voluntary agency, social services or health staff. Funding for schemes is complex and often precarious, dependent on a variety of capital and revenue sources. This is currently being simplified with a single pot of money being made available for intensive management and support needs (see DSS 1998).

Recently the RSLs programme of supported housing has declined, reflecting a shift of emphasis away from special schemes towards the use of independent accommodation with peripatetic or 'floating' support. There are a number of arguments for and against each form of provision.

Arguments for supported housing schemes:

- more likely to ensure long-term provision
- easier to co-ordinate support packages and avoid duplication
- use specialist knowledge and training
- ensure suitable accommodation
- avoid a concentration of vulnerable people in poor-quality areas
- reduce the burden on ordinary housing management

Arguments for floating support:

- does not segregate, label or stigmatize residents
- meets specific needs of each individual
- flexible to meet changing needs
- does not force people to move to get increased or decreased level of support
- no problem of 'silting up' due to lack of accommodation for people to move into
- most people prefer to live in ordinary housing

While there are strong arguments in favour of making more use of floating support and restricting special-needs housing to those with the most complex needs, in reality floating support can easily fail. Financial constraints on all services, the lack of collaboration between agencies and the constantly changing nature of people's needs make it very difficult to ensure continuous adequate levels of support to people in their own homes. Housing managers often feel they are left 'holding the baby' when floating support fails, as discussed below. Vulnerable people need a fully integrated and secure housing and welfare package provided by housing, health and social services agencies working together.

Access to suitable housing

Poor health limits housing opportunities and those in the worst health struggle to gain access to decent housing. Those with ill-health have limited earning capacity and can only afford the poorest quality private housing, and are therefore often dependent on social housing. Following the 1996 Housing Act local authorities are required to give re-housing priority to certain groups including households who need accommodation on medical or welfare grounds and vulnerable homeless people.

Social landlords have always operated some kind of medical priority system. As the expansion of social housing has declined and demand for re-housing on grounds of ill-health has risen, medical priority systems are under increasing pressure. Many GPs are asked by patients to write letters in support of their application and most medical priority systems involve medical staff such as doctors or occupational therapists. However, their knowledge and understanding of the local housing system and what is available is often limited, leading to demands which cannot be met. Priority systems are inherently discretionary with each area determining what kinds of needs are recognized and there is often a tendency to focus on the medical condition rather than on making an assessment of the benefit of re-housing. Proximity to carers is often not taken into account, neither is the alternative of providing aids and adaptations in the existing home. Many local authorities are reviewing their medical priority system and there is great scope for this to be more closely related to community care assessments.

Homeless vulnerable people often have a variety of problems and need a combination of secure, healthy housing plus support to maintain their tenancy. In addition to the problems of providing suitable accommodation discussed on page 103, it is also often difficult to arrange the necessary support. Agencies such as social services, health authorities, probation and voluntary organizations have to be involved and a co-ordinated package of housing and support secured. Some homeless sections of housing departments employ specialized staff such as mental health workers to assess people and arrange support. The need for close inter-agency collaboration is discussed on page 110.

The increasing need for homes suitable for people with mobility difficulties is discussed on page 99. The quality of local information on both what people need and what housing is available is generally poor. A number of local agencies have been established to co-ordinate needs and accommodation, and these are known as disability housing services. They may be linked to a housing association or be independent. Most employ occupational therapists to register and assess individual needs, help with getting adaptations, keep a database of specially designed or adapted housing and match this to needs. This provides a one-stop shop for disabled people, speeds up the adaptation and re-housing process and provides a better fit of property to people. In some areas housing authorities directly employ occupational therapists to assess needs.

Housing agencies have nomination agreements with voluntary organizations, social services and others that can gain priority for someone in need. It is increasingly recognized that housing staff also need to be involved in assessments by other services. Community care assessments and hospital discharge procedures should routinely include housing officers who know what accommodation is available. Similarly the operation of the Children Act needs to be co-ordinated with the assessment and re-housing of very young homeless vulnerable people. Other agencies such as probation, the police and education also need to be involved where appropriate. Matching vulnerable people to property requires effective joint working arrangements between all the relevant services.

Housing management and support

A significant proportion of tenants living in ordinary council and association housing need some form of support. For some, particularly single homeless and very young people, it might be necessary only for a limited time to help with settling in, including help getting furniture and household goods and advice on benefit claims, household budgeting, housekeeping and daily living skills. Many vulnerable tenants also need long-term support to maintain their independence and prevent crises, including emotional support, personal and medical care.

The social role of housing management may be seen as falling along a continuum:

- Core housing management tasks: allocations, rent collection, repairs, enforcing tenancy conditions.
- Intensive management and advice: additional guidance on maintaining a tenancy for vulnerable tenants, housing and welfare benefits, getting a transfer or adaptations, keeping an eye on the tenant, dealing with neighbour problems.
- Dwelling-related support: redecoration, providing furniture, emergency cleaning or rubbish clearance.
- Community support: tenant groups, crime prevention schemes, estate regeneration schemes.
- Brokerage tasks: ensuring that tenants receive services from other agencies such as social services and health, advocating for tenants, involvement in assessments for community care, children at risk.
- Personal support: befriending, shopping, meals, medication, bathing.

(based on Clapham and Franklin 1994)

The Housing Corporation provides the Supported Housing Management Grant for more intensive management for tenants with specific needs, but this is restricted to action which maintains the tenancy rather than more caring personal support.

There is no consensus about where along this continuum the limits of housing management lie, and in practice managers become involved in all of these tasks from time to time. Many vulnerable tenants who need medium and low levels of personal support and some with greater needs are not getting it. Housing managers, including wardens and caretakers, are acutely aware of this and are often forced to step in. However, while they are increasingly called upon to adopt a more caring welfare role towards their tenants, they are also under strong pressures to limit their work to dealing with bricks and mortar (see p. 120).

Ordinary housing managers can only provide restricted help because they do not have the training, time or funding needed to give adequate support. A few social landlords have found the resources to employ specialist workers whose role spans housing management and support.

Housing and community care

While the idea of reducing the use of hospitals and residential institutions initially developed in the 1950s, by the late 1980s the provision of alternative community settings was found to be inadequate, fragmented and chaotic. This led to the passing of the 1990 Health Services and Community Care Act that gave local authority social service departments responsibility to provide a coherent community care service.

Where housing was considered at all, it was seen in a limited bricks and mortar role of providing accommodation and adaptations. However, after the implementation of the provisions DOE/DOH Circular 10/92 *Housing and Community Care* acknowledged that 'adequate housing ... is often the key to independent living' and stressed the need for collaboration with housing agencies. Subsequently there has been a growing recognition of the importance of providing suitable housing, securing access to housing and giving management support.

The community care policy now calls for housing to have input at all levels: strategic planning, assessing needs, and joint working to deliver services. Social services departments have a statutory duty to consult other agencies including housing in the preparation of their community care plans. However, effective strategic planning should involve the co-ordination of all agencies including housing, health, and social services. This is often made more complex where agencies operate at different levels (district and county) and boundaries do not coincide.

In some areas Housing Consortia have been developed – voluntary bodies bringing together all the relevant local agencies to co-ordinate the planning and provision of services, create a joint budget for capital and revenue funding and pool knowledge, skills and expertise. In each case one agency takes the lead and the extent to which others are involved varies.

INTER-AGENCY WORKING TO DELIVER SERVICES

In addition to the specific requirements of the community care programme, agencies need to work together to deliver appropriate services to all those with housing, health and care needs. A key part of every housing manager's work is to liaise with front-line staff in other agencies, including social workers, environmental health staff, health visitors, community psychiatric nurses, hospitals, probation officers and many others in both statutory and voluntary agencies.

However, despite well-intentioned statements at strategic level, inter-agency collaboration is poorly developed overall, and the impressive examples of housing agencies working closely with others are the exception rather than the rule. There are also gaps between the services of different agencies.

Reasons for the lack of successful inter-agency arrangements are:

- shortage of resources
- competition created by the introduction of markets into social welfare provision
- uncoordinated and at times contradictory government policies and programmes
- lack of understanding of the roles and responsibilities of other agencies and false expectations
- poor communication between different organizations with little sharing of information and even distrust.

Effective liaison between front-line staff in different agencies requires both formal structures and informal links, together with:

- formal support and commitment from senior management
- clear understanding of each agency's boundaries of operation
- clear recognition of each worker's roles and responsibilities.

Some local authorities have combined their housing and social services departments. This is only effective where working links are forged at all levels including between housing managers and social workers. Joint local offices can help to provide co-ordinated services by offering a one-stop shop and bringing staff together.

New forms of collaboration are emerging and there are some innovative examples, but experience is patchy and agencies have been working without an overall policy framework at central government level. The Labour government elected in 1997 has recognized the need for a co-ordinated central government approach to community care and initiated proposals for a more integrated approach. The various new action zones, including health action zones, set a model for inter-agency working, especially as they involve pooling budgets between agencies. This may help local organizations to achieve more effective inter-agency collaboration on the ground.

Proposals for reform

The complexities of funding support for those with special needs and the difficulties encountered in inter-agency working have been recognized for some time. The December 1998 DSS consultation document (*Supporting People: A new policy and funding framework for support services*) seeks to address both issues.

In outline, the document suggests the merging of existing funding for the intensive management and support of special-needs groups. The local authority will be under a statutory obligation to provide for the support needs of the community as a whole irrespective of tenure. This would be achieved by a Commissioning Committee composed of representatives of housing, social services and probation, who will be obliged to co-operate, on pain of losing a percentage of the grant.

While the main thrust of the proposals is to be welcomed, the absence of any representation from RSLs or the Housing Corporation on the Commissioning Committee causes concern. Groups traditionally championed by RSLs may miss out, with funds being spread more thinly and made subject to means testing. Some of these concerns may be addressed through the consultation process, but it seems unlikely that any more money will be forthcoming for this group as a whole.

KEY POINTS

- Housing policies arose out of a concern with health, but housing and health policies then diverged during the twentieth century. There is now a renewed awareness of the fundamental links between them.
- Different groups of people have particular housing and health needs. Homeless people experience particularly severe physical and mental health problems yet have very poor access to health services.
- Social landlords aim to give priority to vulnerable people in their allocation systems and provide specialized accommodation including sheltered housing, homes designed or adapted for disabled people, hostels and supported housing. The role of specialized housing is being questioned and there is often little relationship between the local supply and local needs.
- Housing has only recently been recognized as essential to community care. Housing should have an input in strategic planning, in joint assessments of need and in joint working to deliver services.
- Inter-agency collaboration is poorly developed on the ground and needs both formal structures and informal working links, backed up by a co-ordinated government policy framework.
- Proposals to simplify the funding of intensive management and support and to encourage inter-agency working are to be welcomed, but there is no indication of additional funding and there is a risk of some groups being marginalized.

GUIDE TO FURTHER READING

For a general discussion of the links between housing and health, see:
Ineichen, B. (1993). *Homes and Health.* London: E and FN Spon.
For a discussion of housing and other issues facing those with a physical disability, see:
Morris, J. (1990) *Our Homes our Rights: Housing, independent living and physically disabled people.* London: Shelter.
For an excellent practitioner's guide to the nature of mental health problems and the service provision available for this special needs group, see:
Thompson, K., Phelan, M., Strathdee, G. and Shiress, D. (1995) *Mental Health Care: A guide for housing workers.* London: The Mental Health Foundation.

Housing as
as a service

Outline
This chapter discusses the housing service delivered by local authorities and registered social landlords (RSLs). It starts by examining the origins and development of the housing profession. It then focuses on the functions carried out by social housing landlords, highlighting fundamental questions about the proper role of social landlords and whether they should become involved in the welfare of tenants or restrict their concerns to managing the property. As the nature of the housing service has become more complex, it has become essential for housing managers to work in partnership with other agencies. It is now recognized that tenants should be key partners. The final section examines the statutory rights of tenants and their participation in the management of their homes.

ORIGINS AND DEVELOPMENT OF THE HOUSING PROFESSION

The origins of housing management as a profession can be traced back to the 1860s, to a young woman called Octavia Hill. She believed that if tenants were helped with their problems they would then pay the rent and take care of the property, while landlords could provide decent accommodation and still be sure of a 5% return on their capital investment. Her revolutionary approach to the relationship between landlord and tenant involved getting to know tenants and giving advice on housekeeping, hygiene, household budgeting, morals and sobriety. In return the landlord would keep the property in good repair. The emerging housing associations and charities adopted her successful approach. They initially used 'lady volunteers' and then later paid trained middle-class women to manage tenants, collect rents and arrange repairs and maintenance.

However, when council housing developed after the First World War this staff-intensive, social welfare approach was not necessary. The new council tenants were carefully selected, skilled working-class families posing few management problems. Management focused on collecting rents and maintaining the properties. These tasks did not require the sensibilities of the Octavia Hill tradition and were predominantly carried out by men with technical skills in accountancy, public health, surveying, valuation or engineering. The service was fragmented between departments such as Town Clerks and Engineers.

The Octavia Hill method of housing management continued on a small scale. In the 1930s, when councils began to re-house the poorest households displaced by slum clearance, a few authorities recognized the need for more intensive management and employed estate managers. However, in the 1950s, as council housing focused its allocations upon general needs, intensive housing management was again not seen as essential and few women housing managers were employed.

Throughout these years the emerging housing profession was split between two bodies as is shown in Table 6.1.

Table 6.1 The growth of the housing profession

The Octavia Hill welfare approach	The local authority technical approach
1916 The Society of Women Housing Workers formed **1932** The society was expanded to become **The Society of Women Housing Estate Managers** **1948** The society was renamed the **Society of Housing Managers** with entry examinations and for the first time men were admitted	**1931 The Institute of Municipal Estate Managers** worked with the Royal Institute of Chartered Surveyors to introduce a professional examination: the Housing Managers Certificate
1965 The two rival organizations merged and the **Chartered Institute of Housing** was formed	
1999 The Institute of Rent Officers merged with the Chartered Institute of Housing	

The Chartered Institute of Housing (CIH) grew in membership and influence in the 1990s. It gained its Royal Charter in 1984 and now has about 15,000 members. In addition to membership in the UK, the institute has a thriving branch in Hong Kong and an accredited training course in Australia. The professional qualification includes an academic and a work-based element, and, depending on experience, takes two to six years to complete. Most housing officers gain their professional qualification while working in a housing job, but some take a taught full-time or part-time course that is professionally accredited. Universities and colleges of further and higher education provide NVQ/SVQ, BTEC, undergraduate and postgraduate housing education. The proportion of housing workers who are professionally qualified is still under 10% but is rising.

The development of the housing profession highlights the tension between housing management as a technical function focusing on property and housing management as a social function focusing on the welfare of the tenants. When the focus of council activity was on building for general needs in the 1920s, 1950s and 1960s, the technical role was paramount. Since then, new building activity has declined and as the sector has become residualized (see pp. 72–74) and local authorities and RSLs have re-housed increasing proportions of vulnerable tenants. As in the 1930s, this has resulted in the need for more intensive housing management. At the same time, the drive for efficiency and market testing is putting pressure on budgets and making sensitive management more difficult to provide.

The housing profession has long had low status relative to other professional groups. Even recently many senior posts have been occupied by those with other professional backgrounds, for an example see *Housing background not essential*, below.

Housing background not essential

A Chief Housing Officer post in a large metropolitan borough was advertised in 1998 with the words 'Whilst a housing background would be an advantage, it is not essential if you have a proven track record of delivering results from a senior management position in Local Government or similar public service'.

(*Inside Housing*, 9 April 1998)

There is a number of reasons for the low profile of the housing profession:

- Unlike other branches of the welfare state, such as health and education, state housing is not universal.
- Housing provision is dominated by the private sector.
- Social housing caters for a minority of the population, generally the economically weak and marginalized, with little political influence.
- The housing profession does not lobby on behalf of powerful groups in society.
- At the local level, councillors have always been more involved in the detailed operation of the housing service than in other spheres, leaving less discretion to the professional officers.

The history of the development of the housing profession highlights the position of housing at the junction of a number of professional interests and it has been difficult to create clear ownership of a body of skills and knowledge. Issues which are outside the competence of other professions, such as managing housing stock, are not seen to have professional mystique or require a special set of skills. After all, private owners and landlords perform these tasks and there has been virtually no public or academic interest in how the private sector is managed.

However, the management of the public sector is a major activity. There are still over four million council properties in the UK worth an estimated £130 billion, housing nine million people. Managing and maintaining this stock costs over £1.25 billion a year. Nearly 150,000 people are employed in housing, half in local authorities and the rest in associations and the private sector. Those who work in housing must combine the attributes, skills and knowledge of many other professions – technical, managerial and social. This makes housing a complex profession.

AGENCIES WHICH OWN AND MANAGE SOCIAL HOUSING

These agencies are primarily:

- local authorities
- registered social landlords (RSLs).

Local authorities

During the twentieth century every council in the country built and let housing, ranging from a few hundred to over 100,000 dwellings. In addition to building and managing housing for rent, councils have a responsibility to assess local housing needs, respond to homelessness and provide housing advice services. Housing legislation has traditionally been permissive and left local authorities with scope for interpretation, but in the 1980s and 1990s government intervention gradually increased.

Local authorities have been encouraged to consider abandoning their role as landlords altogether by becoming 'enablers', with an emphasis on overseeing local housing provision by other agencies. This new direction opened up the way for local authorities to transfer their housing stock to other agencies, predominantly to RSLs (see pp. 32–35). Since the late 1980s, over 60 authorities have transferred their permanent housing stock and rely entirely on RSLs and other agencies to meet local housing needs.

All housing authorities, including those with no housing stock, are responsible for maintaining a Housing Register and for statutory homeless provisions, if necessary by nomination arrangements with other landlords. They must produce an annual Local Housing Strategy Statement and Housing Investment Plan, a rolling three-year programme presented to the government office for the region. The strategy identifies local housing needs, considers policies for all housing tenures in the area, including enforcing standards in private rented housing, and makes a bid for capital expenditure approval. Housing authorities are encouraged to place the housing role within the wider policy context. This includes identifying relationships with other local programmes like community care, forging links with local agencies such as health authorities and the police, and developing the role of housing in other local strategies, including anti-poverty programmes, regeneration projects and projects to combat social exclusion, local employment and training initiatives, and joint ventures and partnerships. This role requires close working relationships with other departments and agencies (see p. 35).

Registered Social Landlords (RSLs)

RSLs are registered, supervised and regulated by the Housing Corporation, a quango under the direction of the Secretary of State for the Environment, who appoints all its members. The corporation makes grants to RSLs, issues circulars on conduct, has extensive powers of supervision and may remove or suspend from office any management committee member or de-register an RSL.

As RSLs grow in size and importance, there is concern about the way they are governed. The task of the voluntary management committee members has become more onerous. Committees need people with expertise in the complexities of housing finance and also people who can represent the tenants or the locality, and they are having difficulties in finding suitable candidates. Most RSLs are represented by the National Housing Federation, a voluntary organization that acts on behalf of their interests, provides advice and conducts research.

THE FUNCTIONS OF SOCIAL HOUSING LANDLORDS

The following functions of social housing landlords will be considered in turn:

- housing management
- allocation of social housing
- collecting rents
- repairs and maintenance
- dealing with empty property
- dealing with neighbour relationships
- equal opportunities in housing
- aid and advice services.

The role and quality of housing management

For most of the history of state housing, the emphasis has been on expanding the housing stock with little attention paid to the quality of management. By the early 1980s, however, there was pressure to improve housing management from both the right and the left of the political spectrum. The Conservative government was anxious to end the monopoly role of local authorities and reduce expenditure, and labelled council housing as wasteful, inefficient and mismanaged. At the same time, many on the left identified traditional housing management as oppressive, autocratic, remote and paternalistic, with little tenant involvement.

The focus on management standards has led to attempts to improve service standards. Management information systems have been improved with greater use of integrated IT systems.

Staff training and tenant involvement has increased. These local measures have been boosted by government intervention. Authorities must now publish annually about 50 performance indicators covering repairs, rents, lettings, voids, staffing and costs. The Chartered Institute of Housing has produced *The Housing Management Standards Manual*, which provides a benchmark for a range of management and maintenance services (Chartered Institute of Housing 1995). There has been a gradual adoption of quality management approaches, such as quality assurance and customer care. Increasing numbers of social landlords are applying for accreditation for specific management and maintenance functions under the British Standards Council BS5750, which attests that the systems can be relied upon to deliver a specified level of service, or for the Charter Mark under the Citizen's Charter initiative.

CCT and Best Value Programmes

Following on from the privatization of council housing by selling it to other landlords, in the early 1990s the management of the council stock was also opened up to market competition through the introduction of Compulsory Competitive Tendering (CCT) for council housing management. Since 1994, CCT has been phased in to all but the smallest authorities. It requires authorities to divide housing functions between two key roles, 'client' and 'contractor'. Individual contracts drawn up by the 'client' specify what tasks the 'contractor' must undertake.

CCT has brought benefits and incurred costs. Its benefits include the requirement that authorities define their policies, procedures and standards more clearly; and it has tightened up the operation of their functions. It has driven the development of integrated comprehensive IT systems in housing management and, most importantly, it has given a specified role to tenants, who have been defined as 'customers' and given rights to be consulted on the level of services in the contract specification, the selection of contractors and monitoring performance.

On the other hand, CCT has proved very costly and bureau-cratic. Large sums of money have been spent on preparing for it even where there has been no external competition. These costs have had to be found from the Housing Revenue Account and borne by the tenants themselves. Housing officers have become demoralized and there are fears that the drive for economy and efficiency has jeopardized the quality of the service offered.

Many professionals welcomed the announcement in November 1998 that CCT was to be phased out by April 2000, to be replaced by Best Value Programmes. In future all local authorities will produce annual Local Performance Plans, which will identify how housing services are to be improved, including:

- housing repair and maintenance
- community care
- hostel and sheltered housing provisions
- special needs housing
- re-housing services
- private sector renewal
- tenancy relations services
- HMOs
- Housing Benefit
- rent collection.

There will be no requirement for authorities to put services out to competition, but comparing performance and cost with other similar landlords through market testing and benchmarking is seen as essential to achieving Best Value. The Local Government (Best Value and Capping) Bill contains proposals to introduce wide powers for ministers to intervene in 'failing' local authorities. Social landlords will also be subjected to regular inspections by District Auditors and the national Housing Inspectorate, which will be run by the Audit Commission. A direct input from tenants will be required, with all councils expected to introduce council-wide and neighbourhood-level tenant participation compacts by April 2000 (see p. 111).

Financial pressures

The limits to the role of housing management have also been challenged by the financial regime for council housing introduced in the 1989 Local Government and Housing Act, which tightened controls on Housing Revenue Accounts. The links between what tenants pay and the service they get have been highlighted, raising the question of how far the caring role involved in housing management should be paid for out of the Housing Revenue Account.

All these developments have tended to tighten up the definitions of housing management tasks. This has taken place in the context of increasing financial constraints, leading to pressure for the role to be more narrowly defined and pinned down to tangible, measurable activities related to the management of the property. Ironically, at the same time, the residualization of the social housing sector, increasing concentrations of vulnerable tenants, the care in the community policy and the rising numbers of frail older people have resulted in greater need for a more caring role for housing management (see pp. 109–110).

Allocation of social housing

Access and allocation policies are about the rationing of a resource and are controversial. Local authorities have a long-standing obligation to house those most in need, although there has been enormous discretion about how 'need' is defined.

Authorities may set their own restrictions on who is eligible for re-housing. Most do not consider those without a local connection, below 18 years, former tenants with a history of rent arrears or anti-social behaviour or those with other housing alternatives. Many others exclude owner-occupiers, those who are adequately housed and those with an income or capital over a certain limit. Existing tenants wanting to transfer are often ineligible if they have rent arrears, have lived there for less than a certain minimum period, have not kept the property in good condition or have breached the tenancy conditions.

Since the 1996 Housing Act (for Scotland the 1987 Housing (Scotland) Act) local authorities must keep a Housing Register for anyone wanting to be considered for a council tenancy. The register also lists existing tenants who wish to transfer or need to move in order for their home to be modernized or demolished. Both new and existing tenants are in competition for the available property. Across England and Wales, between a quarter and a third of all lettings are made to existing tenants. Of the rest, just under a third are let to those who have been homeless. The proportions vary a great deal and in some areas the homeless take a far higher proportion of lettings, putting pressure on the rest of the Housing Register.

RSLs are not restricted by the 1996 Housing Act and are free to determine their own allocations systems. Many RSLs were established to cater for a specific group such as older people, and only have property suitable for that group. Applicants are normally prioritized using a points system. In addition to nominations from local authorities, many specialist RSLs also have nomination arrangements with local agencies which work with certain groups, for example young vulnerable people or those with mental health problems. RSLs also have to cater for existing tenants transferring and those who need to move as their property is renovated. In some areas local authorities and RSLs are developing common Housing Registers with shared application forms, but applicants are still ranked according to each organization's priority system.

The lettings process involves matching a property to an individual applicant. At this point there is a lot of discretion in the system and the judgement of lettings officers is crucial. They may steer certain households into certain properties and decide who is most deserving or who would fit in where. This is the point at which many investigations by the Commission for Racial Equality (CRE) have uncovered racism, and the factors affecting allocations to ethnic minority households are discussed below (see pp. 129–131). The lettings process also acts as a filtering system, whereby those most desperate for re-housing are likely to be made offers of the poorest quality housing on the assumption that they will accept anything, whereas those in less severe need can be more choosy and wait for a better offer. This is often formalized by allowing only one offer of property to a homeless household, while other categories are entitled to more offers. Table 6.2 shows some of the different objectives and inherent conflicts in the access and allocation process.

Table 6.2 Different objectives and inherent conflicts in the access and allocation process

Allocations objectives	Inherent conflicts in allocations
• meeting house needs • addressing the preferences of applicants • considering the views of the local community • promoting sustainable, conflict-free neighbourhoods • managing the housing stock in an efficient and effective way	• avoiding management problems can be discriminatory • the more choice applicants are given the slower the process will be and the greater the number of empty properties awaiting letting • if the desires of the local community are taken into account this may discriminate against certain groups

Local letting schemes

Both local authorities and RSLs have experimented with local lettings schemes for specific estates which are difficult to let or have particularly difficult management problems. These schemes aim to counter the effects of residualization and achieve a wider social mix by creating more balanced communities (see p. 86). Schemes often restrict lettings to local people and those with links and commitment to the area, limit lettings to families with children, exclude those with a history of anti-social behaviour or aim to attract new groups into social renting – such as young working households or students. Local lettings schemes explicitly do not attempt to meet the most serious housing needs and overtly discriminate against certain household types. They need to be carefully managed to ensure this does not become directly or indirectly racist. Experience suggests that the effectiveness of local lettings schemes is limited and this may be because the problems of these estates originate in the wider economic and social environment. Other ways of sustaining and enhancing communities may be more successful (see pp. 54–58).

Exclusion lists

The growth of exclusion lists has also been controversial. While authorities and RSLs have always had discretion to restrict eligibility for re-housing, the 1996 Housing Act has given backing for formal exclusion lists to be drawn up. It has been estimated that as many as 200,000 households are excluded from access to social housing (Shelter 1998). The lists generally exclude households with a history of anti-social behaviour, rent arrears or criminal convictions. This raises the question of who defines anti-social behaviour and opens up the scope for discrimination. There is also a danger that exclusions may disproportionately affect homeless households and those who do not fit society's norms, such as travellers. Local RSLs and even some private landlords may also refuse to consider anyone on the council's exclusion list. One especially controversial aspect of exclusion is that many schemes specifically cite sex offenders and reinforce the tendency for them to be driven underground, where they may pose an even greater risk to society.

The growth of exclusion lists represents a departure from the role of councils as a safety net for those in most need, and reflects the general concern with law and order and social control.

Collecting rents

Collecting rent is one of the core activities of any landlord. Council and RSL tenants can pay their rent in a number of ways:

- at the local housing office
- at the post office
- through door-to-door collections
- using a bank standing order or direct debit.

Rent arrears

The level of rent arrears is a key performance indicator, and social landlords are under pressure to take prompt action on arrears. At any one time, about a third of tenants have missed one or two payments and are up to four weeks behind with the rent and a further one in seven are in greater arrears. However, much of this could be accounted for by late payment of Housing Benefit and use of direct debit rather than tenants not paying. Arrears figures are also inflated by the debts of former tenants who have left without clearing their account. The real problem of current tenants deliberately withholding rent is therefore much smaller but is difficult to estimate.

Housing Benefit

The present Housing Benefit scheme was introduced in 1988 to provide help to low-income tenants with rental payments. The scheme is administered by local authorities, usually by the city treasury or finance department on behalf of central government. Council tenants receive a housing rebate so they have less or no rent to pay, while housing association and private tenants receive an allowance which is a direct cash payment made either to the tenants or to the landlord. It is estimated that approximately two out of every three local authority and RSL tenants are in receipt of Housing Benefit, with the level of claims even higher among new tenants. For example, in new RSL properties with high rent levels, as many as four out of five tenants have been found to be claiming Housing Benefit (Gray *et al.* 1994).

There are numerous rules determining eligibility for Housing Benefit. Since April 1988 there have been over 125 sets of amendments to the rules. As a result, the scheme is both expensive to administer because of the complexity of the calculation required, and difficult for claimants to understand. Every small change in claimants' personal circumstances must be reported. There are often considerable delays in making Housing Benefit payments and in some authorities there are claim backlogs of more than two months. Such delays have a knock-on effect in terms of increasing rent arrears. A further problem associated with the current system is the low level of take-up of the benefit. In 1993 around 17% of eligible households failed to claim approximately £900 million of Housing Benefit.

Repairs and maintenance

Tenants' satisfaction with housing is closely related to their satisfaction with the repairs service. Social landlords therefore have a strong incentive for carrying out this function effectively. The work needed covers both day-to-day repairs and planned maintenance programmes, such as external repainting and renewing windows and roofs.

The repairs and maintenance service must comply with the landlord's legal duties relating to the condition of the property, and aim to minimize re-let times and empty property, while maximizing the useful life of the housing stock. Social landlords must inform tenants of both the landlord's and the tenant's repair obligations and many landlords publicize target response times for carrying out different repairs according to their urgency.

The structure of the repairs service varies. Some social landlords have a centralized service with the benefits of economies of scale and the ability to employ more specialist workers, while others have a decentralized service which relies on multi-skilled workers who are familiar with the property in the area. Experience suggests that smaller area or estate teams are more efficient than a centralized service.

It is estimated that the local authority sector has a backlog of repairs worth £20 billion. Authorities have increased their expenditure on repairs and maintenance but have failed to keep pace with deterioration. Some tenants carry out a significant amount of repairs, but many are not in a position either to do or to pay for such work. A high proportion of complaints to the Ombudsman concern repairs. The law relating to repairing obligations is complex and involves both civil and criminal law.

Cleaning and caretaking on estates is a basic part of the repair and maintenance service. Other departments or agencies carry out some functions such as regular refuse collection and street lighting, so good liaison is important. The involvement and support of tenants is also vital and some landlords have developed estate agreements which spell out the level of service which should be achieved. Central to this is the role of caretakers. This varies a great deal, from non-resident teams who just clean communal areas, to resident caretakers who take on simple household jobs for residents – such as replacing tap washers and unblocking drains, performing basic housing management tasks or even adopting the role of a 'good neighbour', looking out for frail residents. This enhanced role is referred to as 'caretaking plus' or 'super caretakers' and experiments suggest this provides a cost-effective service. Some social landlords employ a concierge in blocks of flats who is a receptionist and general minder for the block, often operating with a CCTV system. The cleaning and caretaking role is crucial to the appearance of the estate and resident satisfaction.

Dealing with empty property

Social landlords aim to keep empty property to a minimum to maximize rent income, keep up the appearance of estates and minimize the costs of boarding up property. High numbers of empty properties can blight an estate.

It is often difficult to tell when a property is empty. Many tenants have little direct contact with the landlord and may be slow to respond to letters and calls even when rent arrears accrue. Tenants often leave their property without informing the landlord. In some areas there is also a problem of illegal occupancy, where the original tenant has let the dwelling to another person who may be paying the rent but is not entitled to be there. Squatting is less of a problem than in the past.

While social landlords strive to minimize turn-around times between tenancies and void levels are generally low, some have property in need of major renovation which must be empty for long periods.

Unpopular estates and lack of demand

Recently there has been a rise in the number of empty social homes in certain parts of the country. The problem is particularly acute in inner city areas and some RSLs even report problems in letting new homes.

Analysis of social landlords' management of empty property

shows that landlords with more than 5,000 dwellings, particularly those based in the north of the country, have high numbers of empty homes, and it can take a long time to re-let property. The reasons for the difficulties these landlords have in managing voids are complex, but include:

- a fall in the demand for social housing in some areas
- unpopular stock, e.g. bedsit accommodation
- the availability of alternative accommodation, e.g. private rented or cheap private property for sale
- location of social housing on the edge of cities
- high rent levels.

Dealing with neighbour relationships

Neighbour relations have become an increasingly important housing issue in both the public and private sectors. Social housing landlords report they now spend more time dealing with disputes, ranging from trivial to very serious incidents. Anti-social behaviour is generally defined as behaviour that unreasonably interferes with others' rights to use and enjoy their home. This can involve a clash of lifestyle where different social groups have different norms of behaviour. Crime is more specific and disputes commonly relate to drug dealing, assault or burglary. Harassment is defined as behaviour deliberately intended to intimidate or harm an individual or certain group, and includes racial harassment (see p. 130). All these problems are often subsumed under the umbrella term 'nuisance'.

There is a number of reasons why social landlords are increasingly drawn into dealing with neighbour relations. The residualization of the sector has resulted in a concentration of poor and vulnerable tenants into housing which may be high density and poorly designed, often lacks good sound insulation and is inadequately maintained. New tenants are predominantly young households who may have different lifestyles and expectations from the older tenants. The care in the community policy has resulted in more tenants with unconventional behaviour living in ordinary housing, and exacerbated prejudice and fear between neighbours. The drive towards efficiency in the housing service has focused attention on the costs of disputes, including repairs, re-housing, legal costs, loss of income from empty properties and reinforcement of the unpopularity of certain estates.

The most frequent nuisance problem between social tenants is noise, followed by disputes over gardens. Other common issues include verbal abuse, criminal behaviour, harassment, damage to property, dogs, physical intimidation and vehicle repairs. Social landlords use a wide range of measures both to prevent or minimize nuisance and to deal with disputes when they arise.

Under the provisions of the 1996 Housing Act, local authorities may give all new tenants temporary Introductory Tenancies, which after twelve months automatically become Secure Tenancies (see p. 135). This new power has been adopted by a number of authorities, although in practice where tenants are evicted from Introductory Tenancies it is more often for rent arrears than for anti-social behaviour.

Dealing with neighbour disputes requires clear procedures, prompt action and close liaison with other agencies. Some social landlords designate specialist officers to handle conflicts. In many areas there is a mediation service, providing an independent third party which aims to open up channels of communication between the conflicting tenants. This is generally provided by a local voluntary agency and can prevent disputes from escalating. Support for victims is important, especially where there is a threat of violence, and this sometimes involves re-housing. It is also important to work with the perpetrators of anti-social behaviour, especially where they may be vulnerable themselves and in need of guidance and support.

As a last resort councils may use legal action. Injunctions may be sought to prevent someone from causing further nuisance or returning to the property or the locality. This may be backed up by a power of arrest. In addition, landlords can take possession action against tenants who have breached the terms of the tenancy, including involvement in incidents of domestic violence. The legal powers available in Scotland are different, with different statutory grounds for possession and the power to compulsorily transfer a tenant to another property.

As well as these specific housing powers, there is a battery of other powers which can be applied to deal with nuisance, which are not specific to council tenants. Environmental Health powers can be used to deal with Statutory Nuisances including noise, filthy or infested property, the dumping of rubbish, and nuisance by dogs. Other legal powers include the Public Order Act 1986, which makes intentional harassment, alarm or distress a criminal offence; the Noise Act 1996, which creates an offence of causing excessive noise at night; the Protection from Harassment Act 1997, which provides civil and criminal remedies to protect the victims of harassment; and the Crime and Disorder Act 1998, which requires local authorities and the police to work together on local strategies to combat crime and disorder. In addition, the Act introduces court orders to deal with anti-social behaviour, and sets out measures to deal with racially aggravated crime, including racial harassment.

Equal opportunities in housing

Concern with equal opportunities in housing emerged in the 1980s and 1990s. The inherent disadvantages in the housing market experienced by some households are discussed on pages 71–72.

Black and minority ethnic households

Numerous studies and CRE investigations have shown that black and ethnic minority households tend to be allocated the oldest social housing with the poorest amenities, and a disproportionate number of flats rather than houses. This is partly because black households are over-represented among the homeless, and homeless households as a whole tend to be allocated the housing which no one else will take. This is a classic form of indirect discrimination. The common practice of excluding owner-occupiers from eligibility for council housing is another example, which disproportionately affects Asian households living in poor quality homes. In addition some areas do not have sufficiently large homes to meet the needs of some Asian households.

However, not only can such policies have an indirectly detrimental effect on certain household groups, but investigations have also disclosed that black and ethnic minority households can still be treated unfairly in relation to white households in the same position. This often arises from the discretion built into the lettings system in matching applicants to specific homes. The pressure to let empty property quickly and minimize anticipated management problems, and subjective assumptions about what sort of housing would be acceptable and the 'suitability' of a household for a particular area, tend to exclude black households from predominantly white popular suburban estates and confine them to inner city estates. These

129

practices place management objectives above equal opportunities and have unintended effects. However, there is huge scope for more direct discrimination in the lettings system and landlords need to be vigilant. Increasing numbers carry out ethnic monitoring and attempt to deal with any anomalies that are identified.

Racial harassment

Racial harassment can take various forms, ranging from racist graffiti, repeated verbal and written racial abuse and threats, damage to property and arson, to physical assault. Landlords often fail to recognize when a dispute has a racial basis.

Landlords can use the 1997 Protection from Harassment Act which makes intentional harassment illegal and provides some protection for victims of harassment. While these provisions relate to all forms of harassment, new provisions designed specifically to deal with racist crime – including common assault, criminal damage and harassment, alarm and distress – are contained in the Crime and Disorder Act 1998. In addition many social landlords now have a specific clause in the tenancy agreement forbidding racial harassment. Reported cases of racial harassment have risen in the last few years and local studies suggest that there is a high incidence in all areas.

Domestic violence

Dealing with domestic violence should also be the focus of equal opportunity policies in housing services. As landlords, social housing management can support tenants in enforcing the law on domestic violence, but it is generally felt that legal protection is inadequate. Injunctions and exclusion orders are intended to prevent further violence but are difficult to enforce and normally only apply for a maximum of three months. Some social landlords have a clause in the tenancy agreement which prohibits violence and this can be used to evict. Local authorities have a specific duty towards women made homeless as a result of domestic violence, and an increasing proportion of those accepted as homeless have lost their former home through domestic violence. For a further discussion on women's housing needs, see Chapter 4.

The responsibility of social landlords in relation to issues such as racial harassment and domestic violence is sometimes questioned. There are laws designed to protect people in all housing sectors from such incidents and the private sector has no mechanisms for dealing with these issues. Why then should social landlords become involved? This reflects the general debate about the role of social landlords. However, it is generally agreed that as service providers with a social welfare role, social landlords must pay attention to the equal opportunity implications of their functions and this includes the way in which the housing is managed.

Aid and advice services

In the 1980s and 1990s there was a growth in the number of agencies offering specialist housing advice and there are now a wide range of housing advice centres run by both public and voluntary bodies. The type of help offered varies from provision of information to provision of comprehensive advice and advocacy services, including access to legal representation.

Many local authorities provide basic housing advice, a service often combined with the section of the housing department which deals with homelessness. Under the Housing Act 1996 it is a statutory duty for authorities to ensure that advice and information about homelessness is available free of charge to anybody in their area. Authorities can fulfil this duty by giving grants or other support such as accommodation and furniture or by funding workers in local voluntary sector advice agencies. A few authorities have even set up housing advice centres run by advisors who are specialists in housing law, local housing policies and practices, money and debt advice and benefits. In order to avoid a conflict of interest, such centres usually concentrate on providing advice and advocacy to private rented tenants and owner-occupiers rather than council tenants.

There is also a large number of independent advice centres including those run by the Catholic Housing Aid Society. Shelter, the national campaign for the homeless, supports a network of advice centres in conjunction with the National Association of Citizens' Advice Bureaux. A wide range of voluntary agencies provide housing and support, particularly for single homeless people. The type of service provided varies considerably between agencies. Some operate telephone advice services with written self-help packs; others provide more detailed one-to-one advice and advocacy while still others provide services to a particular group of people such as members of ethnic communities. Since

1998 Shelter have run a nation-wide, free 24-hour telephone helpline to provide direct help to people with housing problems.

PARTNERSHIPS WITH OTHER AGENCIES

Local authority housing functions have never been carried out in isolation. Few local authorities have fully comprehensive housing departments and many housing functions such as rent collection, running the capital programme and housing advice are carried out by other council departments. Even where housing services have been run together within one department, there has always been a need to work with others; for example, planners, architects, private builders and developers. Some local authorities devised close working relationships with the private sector during the early 1980s, including private sector building on council land and sales of difficult-to-let blocks of flats to the private sector. Partnerships between the public and private sectors have been further promoted through the Private Finance Initiative.

The 1990s, however, have witnessed a proliferation of the links between housing and other services and agencies. Inter-agency schemes such as community care, regeneration programmes and greater interest in consumer involvement necessitated closer working relationships between agencies. RSLs have become key partners in meeting local housing needs and closer links have been made between local authority housing strategies and the Housing Corporation development programme. In many areas RSLs have become involved in schemes with the private sector to provide property for homeless families.

Increasingly all local government policy initiatives are based on partnerships. The development of the community care policy has brought closer working relationships between housing, health and social services and in some areas consortia have been established to bring local agencies together to provide special-needs housing. RSLs themselves are setting up consortia to generate more favourable financial deals or develop land. The regeneration of housing and urban areas has required organizations to adopted a broader base. Social housing organizations have been encouraged to become involved in local employment and training initiatives; for example, foyer schemes (see p. 105) and the New Deal for the Unemployed, which in addition to assisting unemployed tenants may provide environmental and regeneration schemes on estates or services for vulnerable tenants.

Housing plus

In the late 1990s RSLs began to adopt a 'housing plus' approach to development schemes which incorporate social and economic benefits. The interest in housing plus stems from concerns about the emergence of unpopular, difficult-to-manage RSL estates (see p. 127).

Housing plus schemes normally involve three elements:

1 The physical housing development to be located close to jobs and services, environmentally sensitive with energy-efficient homes, deter crime, and include a community training programme or local labour scheme.
2 Housing management to involve tenant participation and support tenant organizations, and adopt a range of sensitive approaches such as a tailor-made local lettings policy to foster social balance, the involvement of specialists such as youth workers, community safety initiatives, adult training schemes and education.
3 The provision of community facilities to be an integral part of the development such as community buildings, play facilities, crèches, childcare and holiday schemes, youth clubs, sports and games facilities and adult education classes.

There is no specific funding from the Housing Corporation for this approach and RSLs have to find money from a range of sources including the Single Regeneration Budget, European Commission, National Lottery, local authorities and private and charitable sources. They need to develop partnerships with local agencies to harness their activities on an estate.

The housing plus approach goes far beyond traditional housing development and management roles, and sees housing as a potential catalyst for enhancing a range of services. It stresses multi-agency working between housing and a range of social, environmental and economic agencies, and associations may be involved with the local health trust, social services, police, and adult or further education colleges. This mirrors the partnership approach increasingly adopted by local authorities in housing regeneration programmes. However, inter-agency working is often very difficult to achieve in practice.

This review of the development of partnerships reflects the increasing need for housing agencies to work more closely with others. The residualization of social housing has resulted in greater concentrations of vulnerable people who require economic and social support. The rapid administrative changes of the 1980s and 1990s brought a proliferation of agencies in the public, independent and private sectors who had to work together, and resource restrictions that limited what agencies could achieve on their own. Housing managers are particularly aware of the need to work with other agencies because they are often the first to become aware of a crisis in a tenant's life which they are ill-equipped to deal with (see p. 108).

THE ROLE OF TENANTS

This section considers tenancies and rights and also tenant participation.

Tenancies and rights

Tenancy law is complex, reflecting the incremental nature of housing policy. Many social landlords are in favour of a simplification of tenancy law and support a move to a single type of tenancy for all tenants regardless of type of landlord. However, currently there are two main types of tenancies:

- long-term tenancies
- short-term tenancies.

Long-term tenancies

Secure Tenants (Housing Act 1985) include most local authority tenants, those RSL tenants whose tenancy started before 15 January 1989, and New Town Corporation and HAT tenants.
Assured Tenants (Housing Act 1988) include most RSL tenants whose tenancy started on or after 15 January 1989.

Short-term tenancies

Under the Housing Act 1996 local authorities may now grant **Introductory Tenancies** which last for twelve months and subsequently become **Secure Tenancies,** unless the tenant has breached the conditions of the tenancy. Introductory Tenants have fewer rights than Secure Tenants.

Homeless households who are accepted by local authorities and then referred to private rented accommodation are generally given **Assured Shorthold Tenancies** (Housing Act 1988). In exceptional circumstances, RSLs also grant Assured Shorthold Tenancies which provide security for six months, after which the landlord only needs to give two months' notice to the tenant.

Some local authority and association hostels use **Licences** rather than secure tenancies, providing fewer tenancy rights.

Where councils dispose of occupied housing to another landlord, the tenants become Assured Tenants but retain their right to buy. Generally councils and RSLs give joint tenancies to couples or sharing adults.

Secure and Assured Tenants' rights

Secure and Assured Tenants have specific rights, as shown in Table 6.3. For Secure Tenants these are set out mainly in the Housing Act 1985 and are collectively known as The Tenants' Charter. Assured Tenants have fewer rights under the Housing Act 1988 but the Housing Corporation has produced a series of Tenant's Charters which set out additional rights which RSLs are expected to grant (Housing Corporation 1998). These rights are given to tenants of RSLs through their tenancy agreement.

Tenant participation

Having discussed tenants' individual rights, this section now turns to the rights of tenants as a group and their collective involvement in the running of their homes. Throughout history residents have worked together to improve their housing or to fight on housing issues. One example of this form of action is squatting, which has a long tradition and was particularly popular after both world wars. There was a revival in the late 1960s, mostly in empty council property awaiting clearance or renovation. Many of these groups eventually reached agreement with their local authority to remain in the property as short-life housing with some possibility of permanent accommodation. There is also evidence of broader collective action being taken by tenants. The Glasgow rent strike in 1915 and the national campaign against the 1972 Housing Finance Act (see pp. 20–22) are two examples of successful collective protests by tenants. More recently single-issue campaigns have developed concerning tower blocks and dampness. However, given the huge numbers of tenants, especially in the council sector, it is perhaps surprising that they have not used their collective power more frequently.

Table 6.3 Secure and assured tenants' individual rights

SECURE AND ASSURED TENANTS' INDIVIDUAL RIGHTS	
THE RIGHTS	**COMMENT**
Right to buy or acquire	The right to buy is coupled with an entitlement to a discount on the price of the property, which is given on a scale in relation to the length of tenancy. This is repayable on a sliding scale if the property is sold within 3 years.
	The right does not apply to most sheltered or specially adapted housing and the tenancy must be of a minimum of two years.
Right to repair	There are specific time limits for the completion of certain small urgent repair jobs, and if landlords fail to carry out the work within the time limits, tenants can ask for another contractor to be employed to do the repair. Tenants can claim a small compensation for the delay.
Right to improve	Tenants can also improve their dwelling with the landlord's consent, which cannot be unreasonably withheld. The landlord cannot increase the rent as a result, and the tenant can claim compensation for the improvements when finally giving up the tenancy.
Rights to succession	If a Secure Tenant dies, the spouse or a family member who has been living in the property for the last year has the right to take over the tenancy. This right does not include a lesbian partner.
	The legal right to succession to an assured tenancy is limited to the spouse, but the Housing Corporation Tenants' Charter encourages RSLs to extend this to family members in parallel with secure tenancies.
Right to take in lodgers	This right can not be unreasonably withheld.
Right to assign and right to exchange	The right to sublet or assign is subject to complex rules (See Arden and Hunter, 1997).

SECURE AND ASSURED TENANTS' INDIVIDUAL RIGHTS *(cont)*	
THE RIGHTS	COMMENT
Right to information and consultation	Secure Tenants must be given certain information about their tenancy, and local authorities must publish an annual report to the tenants giving specific performance indicators, under the Local Government and Housing Act 1989. The Tenants' Charter requires associations to provide similar information and produce a number of specific annual performance indicators.
Right to be consulted	Secure and Assured Tenants have the right to be consulted about proposed changes to management and maintenance policies and practices.
Right to see tenancy files	Secure and Assured Tenants have the right to see details of the information held about themselves by their landlords.

Recent history has seen a gradual development of opportunities for tenant involvement, often on an estate basis. This can be traced back to the Priority Estates Project (PEP), established by the DOE in 1979. A fundamental principle of the PEP approach was the encouragement of active tenant involvement in the running and improvement of run-down estates.

A further impetus to tenant involvement was given in 1980 when 'independent tenant advice' was successfully launched in Scotland, with the setting up of the Scottish Tenant Participation Advisory Service (TPAS). England followed suit in 1988 when TPAS (England) was set up in with partial funding from the DoE. Both TPAS organizations were given a wide remit to support the development of active participation by tenants and they provide help and advice to landlords and tenants and run consultancy, research and publications services. Partly as a result of PEP and TPAS work, most areas across the country now have local tenant associations. The Tenants and Residents Organization of England acts as a national umbrella organization.

The 1980 Housing Act also boosted tenant groups aspiring to have more involvement in the overall management of housing services by increasing Secure Tenants' rights to 'consultation' with their council landlord. This was further strengthened by new grants established under the 1986 Housing and Planning Act and the 1985 Housing Associations Act. The 1986 Act also paved the way for council tenant management organizations to take over the management of their estates through Estate Management Boards and management co-ops. These are tenant-controlled agencies which employ staff to manage the estate within a set budget, while the council retains ownership and control over allocations and rent levels. The 1993 Leasehold Reform, Housing and Urban Development Act extended this by giving tenants the right to manage their housing, without the initiative having to be taken by the council. There has been limited take-up of these schemes.

The various measures introduced in the late 1980s for the transfer of council housing to other landlords also require the support of tenants, generally through a ballot. This has in fact enabled some tenant groups to reject the government's agenda to shift housing out of council hands, as in the case of Housing Action Trusts, Tenants' Choice and some attempts at voluntary transfer.

It is worth considering why a Conservative government should introduce a set of measures which give tenants more say. The emphasis on market provision redefines the role of tenants as consumers who should be able to exercise choices. This reinforces the undermining of local authority power by providing service users with the ability to take over certain functions or even remove themselves from council control altogether. It can also be seen as part of the desire to make local agencies accountable, and demonstrate efficiency and value for money.

At the same time the political left also supports a greater tenant role, which can be seen as enhancing the power of the working class and making large bureaucracies more accountable. This shows that tenant participation means different things to different people. While tenants may see it as giving them a greater say in decisions, councillors and management board members may see it as helping them to do their job by resolving conflicts and legitimizing decisions, while officers may see it as a way of gaining better information in order to make better decisions. Participation may range from giving information to giving real power, and this is known as the 'ladder of participation' (CIH/TPAS 1989), as shown in Table 6.4.

Table 6.4 The ladder of participation

PROCESS	METHOD	INVOLVEMENT
Tenants decision making	Co-ops/Estate Management Boards	Tenant control
Shared decision making	Tenant representatives on committees/boards	Partnership/delegated power
Bargaining	Discussions with tenants' groups/estate forums/consultative committees	Negotiation
Inviting views	Meetings/talking to tenants' groups	Consultation/dialogue
Seeking information	Questionnaires/polls/surveys/meetings	Public relations
Providing information	Letters/leaflets/newsletters	Information/manipulation

Different actors will want to operate at different rungs on the ladder, but participation will be most effective when all the interest groups are in agreement about the level they are operating at. Experience shows that successful tenant participation also depends upon clear and shared aims, a climate of trust, a willingness to allow decisions to change, and financial and practical support for the tenants. This includes meeting rooms, facilities to produce material, access to information, access to advice, especially on legal and financial matters, and training. It is important for all sides, especially policy makers and landlords, to recognize that tenant involvement and participation is neither a 'quick-fix' nor a panacea for all problems between tenants and landlords. It takes time and a great deal of effort to develop confidence, trust and skills. Many tenant groups develop over a single issue, particularly estate renovation, and may be difficult to sustain after the issue is resolved. A failed participation exercise can cause frustration and disillusionment on all sides and ruin the chance to get tenants involved on another occasion. Therefore tenant involvement in specific housing issues needs to be seen as a part of wider attempts to create sustainable communities.

In the early 1990s about half of local authorities and two-thirds of associations provided some form of support for tenant organizations, such as free or subsidized premises, grants, administrative support, or free or subsidized training. Over a quarter of authorities and fewer associations employed specialist staff to promote tenant participation, while just under a third of social landlords had advisory or consultative committees with tenant membership. Over a third of associations had tenants with full voting rights on the management committee, but local authorities are forbidden from giving voting rights to tenants on the main housing committee under the 1989 Local Government and Housing Act.

Current housing policies enhance the potential role of tenants. The requirements to consult on voluntary transfers, the Single Regeneration Budget, Compulsory Competitive Tendering (CCT) and Best Value have given tenants access to a wealth of information about housing services and costs and established new procedures for tenant involvement. The concern with customer care gives scope for tenants' views to be taken into account, and the London Borough of Kensington and Chelsea has transferred the whole of its housing stock to a tenant-managed organization. Both the DETR and Housing Corporation require housing agencies to demonstrate a systematic approach to participation. Further proposals to involve tenants have been made by the Labour government elected in 1997, which intends to introduce Tenant Compacts in all local authority areas from April 2000. The aim of Tenant Compacts is to improve standards of tenant involvement in service provision across the country. The emphasis is on collective tenant empowerment at the district and more local estate or scheme level. The three key objectives of Tenant Compacts are to:

1 make tenants aware of all the options for involvement in the delivery of housing services
2 provide tenants' groups with the skills and support necessary to choose what level of participation they want
3 provide a flexible framework that allows tenants to increase their involvement where and when they choose.

Experience suggests that only a small minority of tenants become actively involved in participation exercises and there is always a danger that those who do get involved are unrepresentative and unaccountable. Most tenants do not want the responsibility of managing their estate. This may be because they are generally satisfied with the service, are cynical and mistrust the landlord, lack training and confidence, or have too many other commitments to devote time and energy to a greater role. One of the advantages of being a tenant is that the landlord is responsible for the dwelling and this is essential for the increasing numbers of vulnerable social tenants. While tenants should have a clear role in determining what services are provided and how they are delivered, and their views should always be central, the role of a social landlord is to hold the ultimate responsibility.

KEY POINTS

- The development of the housing profession highlights the tension between housing management as a technical function dealing with property, and housing management as a social function dealing with the welfare of the tenants. At different times in history either one function or the other has dominated.
- The housing service is big business, spending about £1.25 billion a year managing and maintaining a stock of four million properties housing nine million people.
- The work of social landlords changed in the 1980s and 1990s with greater central government intervention in management and maintenance, the development of a strategic housing role for local authorities, a reduction in the role of local authorities as landlords and the introduction of competition into management and maintenance activities.
- There has recently been increasing concern about the quality and efficiency of the housing service, coupled with conflicting pressures to adopt either a narrower focus on property or a wider focus on tenant welfare.
- The allocation of housing is controversial, as it involves the rationing of housing to those judged to be most in need and the exclusion of others.
- Social landlords are increasingly drawn into dealing with neighbour relations, reflecting the broader social concern with law and order. This marks a shift towards greater involvement by social landlords with tenant welfare.
- Social landlords need to pay attention to the equal opportunities implications of the service, including the

allocation of housing to different groups, the response to incidents of racial harassment, and the approach to cases of domestic violence.

- There has been a growing focus on partnerships between services and agencies and a recognition of the need to link housing services with broader social and economic programmes, especially for housing regeneration. However, while inter-agency collaboration has developed in certain areas of the housing service, it is not evident in the delivery of day-to-day housing management and maintenance.
- The individual rights of social tenants were enhanced in the 1980s and 1990s. There has also recently been greater scope for tenants to become collectively involved in the management of their housing. This can range from simply giving tenants information to giving tenants real power, but the different actors involved can have different objectives and expectations. While tenants should have a clear role in the housing service, it may be argued that the benefit of being a tenant lies in ultimate responsibility being taken by the landlord.

GUIDE TO FURTHER READING

For a full account of the principal rights and responsibilities of social landlords and their tenants, see:

Arden, A. and Hunter, C. (1997) *Manual of Housing Law.* (Sixth edition). London: Sweet and Maxwell.

Among other topics it covers security of tenure, harassment and illegal eviction, relationship breakdown, disrepair and homelessness. It is designed for practitioners, non-lawyers and students and is easy to use.

For a key introductory text on social housing, see:

Harriott, S. and Matthews, L. (1998) *Social Housing: An introduction.* Harlow: Longman.

It is written by a housing practitioner and a housing lecturer and describes in some depth key management tasks such as housing allocations, collecting rents, managing empty properties and repair strategies.

For an excellent guide to the management of social housing, see:

Pearl, M. (1997) *Social Housing Management: A critical appraisal of housing practice.* London: Macmillan.

It explores the dilemmas, demands and difficulties experienced by housing practitioners. It is clearly written and addresses issues such as the difficulties in managing a residualized stock, the role of tenants, housing professionalism and managing in partnership.

For more detailed information on day-to-day housing management tasks, see:

Chartered Institute of Housing (1995) *The Housing Management Standards Manual.* Second edition. Coventry: Chartered Institute of Housing.

Housing issues for the twenty-first century

7

Outline

This chapter draws upon the analysis of housing in the rest of the book to speculate on issues for the beginning of the twenty-first century. Four broad sets of issues are discussed. These stem from four viewpoints: households and the role of different housing markets, social housing agencies and the role of social housing, the state and the role of the state in housing intervention, and housing professionals and the role of housing policy. The conclusion is that housing must be seen as a key part of wider social, economic and welfare policy and that housing organizations must direct their efforts towards achieving more successful inter-agency collaboration.

THE BIG PICTURE

There is an inherent tension in housing policy between long-term and short-term objectives. This is more marked than in other fields of social policy because housing is particularly inflexible.

- The housing stock is a fixed asset lasting decades and often centuries.
- It takes many years to alter the housing stock significantly, through either the development of new housing or alterations to the existing stock.
- Housing investment depends upon a high level of capital expenditure with a commitment from public and private expenditure plans looking several years ahead.
- The system of housing finance is a major, in-built part of every household's budget as well as of the national economy as a whole; any alterations must be planned and carefully staged to avoid undue disruption.

In contrast to the inherently long-term timescales of housing activity, political decisions are usually geared to the electoral cycle and governments are rarely willing to make decisions which show little benefit in their term of office. There is often a reluctance to make long-term capital investments. On the other hand, capital expenditure can often be cut with little immediate apparent effect, as happened throughout the 1980s and 1990s, despite warnings from the housing profession.

The complexity of housing issues also inhibits radical revision. Housing reflects and affects the economic and social framework in which it is located. Housing is influenced by demographic, economic, fiscal and social trends, while housing policy changes have their own impact on all of these aspects. Programmes designed to deal with one issue often have unintended effects in other fields and it is only too easy for policies to cancel each other out or contradict each other. The major spending reviews and policy commitments of the Labour government elected in 1997 attempted to take a broader approach by developing 'joined-up thinking' around problems of urban policy and social exclusion. It is extremely unlikely that a future package of coherent, rational policies will emerge which can tackle housing problems across the board; there will always be uncertainty and scope for speculation.

Housing experts have not had a good track record of predicting the next policy move, especially in the 1980s and 1990s. The long-term political consensus on housing policy quickly evaporated in the early 1980s, for example, under a government prepared to question long-standing assumptions and goals. Looking into the future is a hazardous exercise, in danger of being rapidly over-taken by events, but any wide-ranging analysis would be incomplete without an attempt to pull out some of the significant threads for the future. Housing debates are beginning to focus on several long-term questions which are predicted to challenge housing policy well into the twenty-first century.

This book has approached housing from historical, political, technical, social and organizational perspectives. This analysis of future trends is derived from the perspectives of the various actors involved in housing – households, social housing agencies, the state and housing professionals – to identify four broad issues.

■ Households are concerned that the housing market meets current and future needs; and is flexible, affordable, accessible, available and provides choice. The issue is the role of different housing markets.

- Social housing agencies are concerned with the future of the sector and in particular for whom it will cater, how it can overcome current problems and how it can best meet current and potential tenants' needs. The issue is the future role of social housing.
- The state is concerned with the appropriate extent of intervention in housing, including how much control should be exercised over social housing tenants, to what extent the state should intervene in the private housing market and the scale of public spending. The issue is the future role of the state.
- Housing professionals are often concerned with the apparent lack of political attention to housing, the erosion of housing as an item of public expenditure and the increasingly uncertain links between housing and the broader welfare agenda. These issues pose questions about the future role of housing policy.

Each of these elements is considered in turn.

THE ROLE OF DIFFERENT HOUSING MARKETS

The development of the housing system in the twentieth century was based on an assumption of stable, predictable household needs, with each sector of the housing market catering for a particular type of household at any one time. Housing policy focused on the development of the public sector, catering for those who needed assistance to obtain a decent home. This derived from the belief that the public sector would break the link between low income and poor housing. This approach underpinned housing policy during a period of tenure adjustment, as the dominance of the private rented market was replaced by the dominance of owner occupation. This process is now virtually complete, yet each tenure no longer fulfils a clear role. This stems from changes in both housing markets and household needs.

Each housing sector no longer caters for a distinct group of households. The owner-occupied market is now heterogeneous, stretching beyond the comfortable middle class, and including large numbers of economically insecure households. The social rented sector has at different times catered for the better-off working class and for the most needy, as discussed in Chapter 2. It has tended to cater for a narrowing range of household types in the process of the residualization of the sector in the 1980s and 1990s. There is growing interest in attempts to alter the profile of new tenants to achieve greater social mix in neighbourhoods and tackle the concentration of social exclusion. At the same time the private rented market has been recognized as having a crucial complementary role to social renting and in some ways the different elements of the rented market have become more interchangeable than before.

Social changes have resulted in less clear-cut household formation. Households are more fluid, with higher rates of divorce and separation, and greater numbers of unmarried couples and lone-parent families. As households form and reform their housing needs change frequently. This process has been coupled with greater job insecurity, leaving more people with varying and unpredictable incomes. Many households, especially in inner urban areas, have become very mobile between tenures, not following a predictable progression from one sector to another. The social rented sector has always assumed that, once a household got to the front of the queue, it would remain in the property for a long period, indeed often until the death of the widowed spouse, perhaps some 40 years later. The sector is therefore finding it difficult to adjust to much more unstable and varying levels of demand – but it is highly unlikely that this pattern will change in the foreseeable future.

This increasing fluidity in both housing demand and household formation makes the traditional assumptions of tenure-based housing policy less appropriate for many reasons:

- Poor households now live in all tenures and move in and out of different sectors more often.
- Housing subsidies have shifted from underpinning production to underpinning consumption, so that finance is determined more by who occupies the property than by ownership *per se*.
- Public and private finance have been mixed to break down divisions in the rented sector, through the use of private finance for housing associations, public support for private renting, the emergence of local housing companies and the increasing interest in the development of partnerships between public and private sector organizations through the Private Finance Initiative.
- Tenure segregation at the neighbourhood level has been altered by the development of mixed tenure estates, through the right to buy, new mixed tenure schemes and the development of shared ownership.
- Traditional political allegiances have become more blurred.

The outgoing Conservative government of the mid-1990s had come to accept limits to the expansion of owner occupation and was reducing the financial support for the sector, while at the same time beginning to recognize a residual role for social renting and a need for limited financial support for private renting. The Labour government elected in 1997 did not dislodge the right to buy and has maintained support for the contribution of private finance, the selective transfer of council estates and the growth of housing companies.

- The assumptions about the continued expansion of owner occupation have had to be abandoned in the face of acknowledged limitations on its growth, so that the sector is predicted to stabilize at no more than 75% of the housing market overall.

As the ownership and financing of housing increasingly straddle the public/private boundary, the focus of housing policy may shift from tenure and adopt a more flexible and pragmatic approach to intervention in different types of housing market. Policies narrowly geared to one tenure are no longer appropriate. This development was anticipated by the 1985 Inquiry into British Housing headed by the Duke of Edinburgh, which took a broad overview of housing policy and promoted a level playing field of housing finance geared to household needs rather than any prescribed pattern of ownership (NFHA 1985).

The challenge for housing policy in the twenty-first century will be to nourish a more flexible and adaptable system, which is more capable of accommodating social, demographic and household life-cycle changes. A relatively tenure-neutral system would provide assistance to households in all sectors as and when it was needed, and give incentives in all sectors for adequate maintenance. This must recognize that an unaided free market cannot provide decent low-cost housing for all, and that a degree of intervention and investment will always be essential.

THE ROLE OF SOCIAL HOUSING

Council housing developed in response to fears of disease, crime, an inadequate labour force and political dissent, as discussed in Chapter 2. It initially housed the better-off working class, and soon catered for the poor as they were re-housed from the slums. In the last few decades, as the sector has gradually become residualized and associated with social, economic and physical problems, council housing has been seen as a problem in itself rather then the solution to a problem. In the 1980s the sale of local authority housing and the privatization of housing associations met relatively little resistance for many reasons.

- There was a lack of a strong professional interest seeking to preserve it, unlike medicine, for example.
- State housing does not have almost universal coverage like state education or health.
- The tenants are generally poor and have little power.
- Society as a whole is no longer threatened by the public health fears of the early twentieth century, which underpinned the creation of social housing.

However, there has more recently been a new appreciation of the need for some kind of social rented sector which has stretched across the political spectrum. This was sparked by the private market boom and bust which exposed the fragility of owner occupation, by the widening gap between rich and poor, and by the process of economic restructuring which has created a permanent pool of unemployed and insecure workers who may never be able to buy their homes. Even so, the precise role of social housing in the twenty-first century is far from clear cut.

Faced with a concentration of social and economic problems in particular neighbourhoods, landlords are increasingly attempting to engineer social mix on estates and mitigate the effects of residualization by departing from rigid policies of allocating according to need. They are selecting and rejecting tenants through greater use of certain strategies.

- Local lettings schemes have been introduced on particular estates or for particular properties.
- Exclusions were legitimized by the 1996 Housing Act.
- Landlords are creating introductory and insecure tenancies. In London about a quarter of all current lettings are not secure, largely due to homeless households, as permitted in the 1996 Act. After the statutory two years many of these will only be granted introductory tenancies, giving these new 'second-class' tenants three years of insecurity in total, and making them especially vulnerable to eviction through rent arrears.
- Landlords may take possession action to evict anti-social tenants and those in rent arrears. The use of this strategy has risen significantly in the past few years.

With groups of people being rejected or given only insecure tenancies in the social rented sector; with household structures becoming more fluid, forming and reforming at a greater rate; and with social rents often rising to a level which is close to private rents, the established distinctions between public and private renting are rapidly changing and households are moving in and out of the two sectors at a greater rate. Net turnover rates in council housing in England have doubled in the 1980s and 1990s, offsetting the one-third reduction in the stock of council homes so that the number of dwellings let to new tenants has been roughly constant. This increase in turnover reflects a growing exodus of council tenants into private rented housing. Movers tend to have been council tenants for less than five years. Many of those moving out plan to return to council renting in future, seeing the sectors as interchangeable. This group may contain a high proportion of households which are splitting up and reforming. Other tenants see private renting as a stepping stone towards owner occupation. This suggests that councils are taking on the role of providing flexible short- to medium-term housing more traditionally associated with the private rented market, placing new demands on tenant management, allocations and the need to tap new sources of demand.

The re-let rate of social housing varies from one area to another and is particularly high in urban and declining industrial areas in the north of England, where it is often associated with abandonment of property, difficult-to-let estates or unpopular property types, such as sheltered housing. In these areas social landlords have to abandon allocation practices geared to rationing and adopt a marketing approach which provides quicker access, responding to demand in a similar way to the private rented sector. There is often also competition from the widespread availability of low-cost owner-occupied dwellings.

The phenomenon of difficult-to-let estates seems to contradict the projected shortfall in social housing, which arises if one compares the estimated need for an additional 60,000–100,000 social rented homes a year up to 2016 against the provision of new lettings at only 40,000 a year. However, housing is immobile and cannot adjust to strong regional disparities in demand, which reflect ever-increasing differences between the economic prospects of different regions. While some areas have more than enough social rented housing, others still have severe shortages.

At the same time the role of the private rented market has changed, increasingly catering for those who are voluntarily moving out of the social rented sector. It is also being used by social landlords to discharge their statutory duties to the homeless by nomination to private lets and the use of various leasing and managing arrangements. The private sector is also the only option for those who are excluded from social renting because they are ineligible, have been evicted or will not live in poor-quality social housing, although this function of taking the 'spill over' from the social sector is limited. The private rented sector is no longer expanding as the housing market recovers – it is generally of poor quality, has high rents, and ready access is hampered by the extent to which prospective tenants need deposits to rent properties. There is also evidence that part of the private market is reluctant to cater for those on Housing Benefit, reflected in a significant decline in the number of private tenants getting benefit, especially since restrictions were introduced in 1996. There may be an emerging group of 'excluded' households which are unable to obtain social housing and are deemed unacceptable by private landlords as well.

These changes in the role of rented housing raise several issues:

- There is no longer an undifferentiated role for social housing – it varies between different parts of the country.
- The high household turnover in social housing is both a symptom and a cause of social disorder, threatening social stability on estates and contributing to social exclusion.
- Social landlords cannot operate in isolation from other services, because for many new tenants re-housing needs to be part of a package of support services for it to be successful.
- As social landlords increasingly abandon their 'safety net' role, by excluding, rejecting or only temporarily housing certain households, there is no sector of the housing market which reliably caters for such households.

THE ROLE OF THE STATE

The state has an established role in the housing system, which has mainly focused on the provision of public housing for those not catered for by the market. The increasing residualization of social renting and the persistence of housing problems in the private sector raises two key questions about the appropriate role of the state in twenty-first-century housing.

The first question concerns the degree of social control which should be exercised within the social rented sector. The residualization of social housing, reflected in a concentration of vulnerable households, including the poor and those with personal problems, has increasingly called for a more interventionist role – whether in the form of additional support for households or of greater social control over tenants. Chapters 5 and 6 have discussed the need for social housing management to adopt a more 'welfarist' role, at the risk of conflicting with a narrower property management perspective.

At the same time the government has created a climate of greater social control in many areas of life, through emphasis on law and order, increasing use of CCTV surveillance in public places and a tightening up of police powers to control the streets. Local authorities have been given more tools of social control over their tenants, as the law enables them formally to exclude certain households, make greater use of eviction for rent arrears, give probationary tenancies, provide only temporary housing for the homeless, devise local letting schemes which exclude certain households, make curfew orders on tenants and develop a more proactive approach to breaches of tenancy conditions – particularly in cases of domestic violence and racial harassment. Housing agencies now have wide scope to intervene in tenants' lives and are becoming powerful agents of social control to an extent which is not applicable to any other housing sector.

The second question concerns the appropriate level of state intervention in private housing. Governments have hesitated to interfere directly in private renting and owner occupation, instead achieving powerful indirect influence through financial measures. Traditionally Conservative governments have sought to minimize intervention while left-wing governments have favoured greater controls, but often this has been more evident in rhetoric than in policy commitments. The nature of the housing market at the end of the twentieth century challenges this traditional role of the state in various ways. First, a substantial number of marginal homeowners are at risk of losing their home, and mortgage interest assistance for those on Income Support is inadequate, prompting a case for introducing compulsory private insurance for all owners.

A second policy dilemma concerns the significant amount of private housing in poor condition in both rented and owned sectors. Proposals for greater local authority powers to enforce conditions in the rented sector have been seen as a threat to landlord incentives and the Labour government elected in 1997 is taking a limited approach to the registration of HMOs where the worst conditions are found. There are growing concerns about the future quality of the national housing stock, particularly in recognition of the costs poor housing imposes on public services such as housing, health and care. Slum clearance programmes are unlikely to be reintroduced in areas of predominantly owner-occupied housing. For several decades the state has intervened on a voluntary basis by providing improvement grants to home-owners and there may be scope for other forms of support in the future, such as providing advice through Home Improvement Agencies or requiring vendors to undertake a survey. However, it is not clear how far the state should become financially involved in the maintenance of private housing, and awkward questions arise about the fairness of the state giving money to an owner who then benefits from an enhanced asset.

Controls over new private building have been exercised largely through the systems of planning and building regulations. This system has failed to ensure an adequate supply of new homes, which may result in high prices, market instability and regional imbalances. Governments have recently encouraged the use of brownfield land for new housing, reducing the dependence on greenfield sites. There are now powers to ensure homes are built to mobility standards through the extension of Building Regulations Part M to many sites. However, regulations do not encourage or enforce environmentally sensitive developments, which minimize the use of non-renewable resources and are environmentally sustainable, despite the existence of government targets to achieve reduced CO_2 emissions necessitating energy efficiency measures in housing.

Many empty homes are privately owned. Local authorities have virtually no powers to bring them back into use. This is especially frustrating in areas of high demand, but levers to intervene no longer exist. A programme taking private housing into public ownership would be both financially and politically inappropriate.

The above issues all challenge the role of the state, presenting arguments for greater intervention into private housing in the wider national interest, at the risk of threatening the traditional freedoms of private owners. A precedent of a kind has been set by the requirement that owners use the asset value of their home to pay for care support under the care in the community programme. However, any government would be very nervous about introducing more controls over what are regarded as the inviolable individual rights of the homeowner.

This hesitancy about intervening in the private housing sector stands in stark contrast to the moves towards greater control of social housing tenants, raising questions about policy consistency and the balance between individual consumer sovereignty and the goals of equity and social justice.

THE ROLE OF HOUSING PROFESSIONALS

The structure of this book shows that housing can be seen from a variety of different perspectives, which leads to both strengths and weaknesses. The strength is the central role of housing to all aspects of social welfare and to the economy. An analysis of housing draws on many other disciplines, making it varied and multi-faceted. On the other hand, there is a lack of a clear and unique body of knowledge which defines housing study. This is illustrated by the uncertainty over the boundaries of housing management discussed in Chapter 6, and the extent to which it should encompass a social welfare role. Housing had a more clearly defined profile when the main activity was new building – a visible public programme with a large budget. Now the social house building programme is at an all-time low, housing is being crowded out by the demands of other services, especially as it has never been defined as a universal right like health or education. As a result, there is a need to rethink the identity of the discipline.

This situation is starkly reflected in the low profile of housing in current political debate. In the 1997 election, for example, the priorities, aims and objectives of the incoming Labour Party were health, crime and justice, welfare, transport, education and the economy, with virtually no mention of housing. How different from the early 1950s, when the main parties vied with each other for the most ambitious targets for new house building.

It is also significant that the levers of housing finance are not controlled by the Minister of Housing.

- Housing Benefit is under the control of the DSS and, because it plays a key role in the whole tax and welfare system, is little influenced by purely housing issues.
- Interest rates, which critically affect all sectors of the housing market, are no longer under direct government control, following the decision of the Blair government in its first week of office to pass the responsibility to the Monetary Committee of the Bank of England.
- Most building societies have acquired PLC status, becoming indistinguishable from banks or insurance companies, and are increasingly focusing on activities other than housing.
- Before it was phased out, MIRAS was the concern of the Inland Revenue, and any adjustments were made by the Chancellor of the Exchequer rather than the Minister of Housing.
- Even the budget over which the DETR has some control is subject to non-housing influences. For revenue, this is intricately linked to Housing Benefit through the system of subsidies to local authorities, while there are proposals to pool all council capital expenditure across departments and abandon an independent capital housing programme.

It could be argued that British housing policy, service delivery and professional practice are adopting a more European profile. Traditionally housing has not been as highly politicized in Europe as in the UK, local authorities do not have distinct housing departments and there is no well-developed housing profession. The social and economic context in many European countries has converged, with growing acceptance of the problems of social exclusion and the need for a multi-agency approach to tackle this. Housing policy is not an area of responsibility of the European Commission, except through the directives on the procurement of building contracts, the construction industry and the environment. However, European social and economic policies do have an effect upon housing policies in member countries by affecting the level of public expenditure, rules for convergence, moves towards the creation of a single market in mortgage finance, the mobility of labour between countries, consumer legislation and employment laws. It is therefore quite plausible to argue that the distinct role of housing which has prevailed in Britain is likely to move gradually towards a more European model, marginalizing its role as a separate area of public policy.

These concerns have generated debates about the future of housing policy. It is increasingly acknowledged that housing policies can only be effective when aligned with other policies such as social welfare, employment, health and education. However, the same can be said of each of these fields, posing challenges to tight demarcations of policy areas and professional boundaries. Those trying to effect change in social care, health, education, crime and employment understand the limits of their effectiveness in the absence of decent housing as a bedrock, while learning how much inadequate housing generates greater costs to these other services. The irony is that while some housing experts are introspectively worrying about whether the discipline has a future, other professions are becoming increasingly aware that housing is crucial. This is reflected in the realm of policy too. The Labour government's approach to social exclusion, for example, gave housing a central place in strategies for neighbourhood renewal (Social Exclusion Unit 1998).

Rather than conducting a sterile debate about the future of housing policy, housing commentators could make a more useful contribution by focusing on the inter-relationships between housing and other services. Social housing will remain a significant tenure, predominantly housing the most needy. Landlords can no longer work in isolation from other social, economic and welfare services. This thread has run throughout this book and points the way to the future. Housing programmes need to be better integrated, agencies need to co-ordinate their work and front-line staff need to develop effective inter-agency collaboration. There is a great deal of useful and creative work going on at the local level, which needs continued support and encouragement. One central ingredient is better knowledge and understanding of other disciplines and services. This book has attempted to make a contribution to this process by providing an introduction to and analysis of the way housing works through the key issues of today and tomorrow.

KEY POINTS

- There is an inherent tension between the inflexibility of the housing system based on a fixed stock of dwellings, and the short-term emphasis of much public policy.

- Predicting trends in housing is notoriously difficult, but four broad sets of issues can be identified which are likely to feature in housing debates in the early twenty-first century.
- The role of each housing sector has changed over the twentieth century, with tenures no longer catering for a distinct group of households and increasing fluidity in both housing sectors and household formation.
- The future role of social housing is uncertain, with social landlords becoming more selective in who they house, greater household movement between social and private renting, significant regional variations in the need for social housing and unresolved questions about who is ultimately responsible for housing the excluded.
- There is a marked contrast between the increasing degree of social control over social sector tenants and the reluctance of the state to intervene in the private housing market, despite problems of supporting marginal homeowners, poor conditions, low new building standards and empty private property.
- Rather than dwell on concerns about the future of housing policy and of the discipline as a whole, it is more fruitful to recognize that housing is a key part of social, economic and welfare policies which calls for more effective collaboration between policies, agencies and professionals.

GUIDE TO FURTHER READING

For a more detailed account of the relationship between recent housing policy and wider social change, including examples of the role of citizenship in housing policy, see contributions in:

Marsh, A. and Mullins, D. (eds) (1998) *Housing and Public Policy: Citizenship, choice and control*. Buckingham: Open University Press.

For commentary and analysis on key housing issues and an outline agenda for future policy development in the twenty-first century, see:

Williams, P (ed.) (1997) *Directions in Housing Policy: Towards sustainable housing policies in the UK*. London: Paul Chapman Publishing.

Sources

LIST OF REFERENCES

Anderson, I., Kemp, P. and Quilgars, D. (1993) *Single Homeless People.* London: HMSO.

Arblaster, L. and Hawtin, M. (1993) *Health, Housing and Social Policy: Homes for wealth or health?* London: Socialist Health Association.

Arden, A. and Hunter, C. (1997) *Homelessness and Allocations.* Fifth edition. London: LAG.

Arden, A. and Hunter, C. (1997) *Manual of Housing Law.* Sixth edition. London: Sweet and Maxwell.

Audit Commission (1998) *Home Alone: The role of housing in community care.* London: Audit Commission.

Audit Commission (1989) *Housing the Homeless: The local authority role.* London: HMSO.

Aughton, H. and Malpass, P. (1994) *Housing Finance: A basic guide.* London: Shelter.

Centrepoint Soho (1996) *The New Picture of Youth Homelessness in Britain.* London: Centrepoint.

Chartered Institute of Housing (1995) *The Housing Management Standards Manual.* Second edition. Coventry: Chartered Institute of Housing.

CIH (1998) *Housing and Health: Good practice briefing issue 13.* Coventry: Chartered Institute of Housing.

CIH/TPAS (1989) *Tenant Participation in Housing Management.* London: Chartered Institute of Housing/TPAS.

Clapham, D. and Franklin, B. (1994) *Housing Management, Community Care and Competitive Tendering. A Good Practice Guide.* Coventry: Institute of Housing.

Conway, J. (ed.) (1988). *Prescription for Poor Health: The crisis for homeless families.* London: SHAC.

Crook, A., Kemp, P., Anderson, I. and Bowmen, S. (1991) *Tax Incentives and the Revival of the Private Rented Sector.* New York: Cloister Press.

Department of the Environment (1995). *Projections of Households in England to 2016.* London: HMSO.

DOE and DETR *Annual Homelessness Statistics.* London: HMSO.

Department of Social Security (1998) *Supporting People: A new policy and funding framework for support services.* London: DSS.

EDAW, Global to Local and De Montfort University (1997) *Living Places: Sustainable homes, sustainable communities.* London: National Housing Forum.

Forrest, R., Murie, A. and Williams, P. (1990) *Home Ownership: Differentiation and fragmentation.* London: Unwin Hyman.

Gibbs, K. and Munro, M. (1991) *Housing Finance in the UK.* Basingstoke: Macmillan Education.

Gilroy, R. and Woods, R. (1994). *Housing Women.* London: Routledge.

Goodchild, B. (1997) *Housing and the Urban Environment: A guide to housing design, renewal and urban planning.* Oxford: Blackwell Science.

Goodwin, J. and Grant, C. (eds) (1997) *Built to Last: Reflections on British housing policy*. Second edition. London: *Roof* Magazine.

Gray, B., Finch, H., Prescott-Clarke, T., Cameron, S., Gilroy, R., Kirby, K. and Mountford, J. (1994) *Rent Arrears in Local Authorities and Housing Associations*. London: HMSO.

Griffiths, D. (1982) 'Triple onslaught on council housing', in *Labour Weekly*, 12 March 1982, p. 6.

Harriott, S. and Matthews, L. (1998) *Social Housing: An introduction*. Harlow: Longman.

Housing Corporation (1998) *Residents' Charter*. London: Housing Corporation.

Ineichen, B. (1993). *Homes and Health*. London: E and FN Spon.

Joseph Rowntree Foundation (1996) *Mixed and Flexible Tenure in Practice: A briefing note from the Joseph Rowntree Foundation*. York: York Publishing Services.

Kemp, P. (1991) 'From solution to problem: council housing and the development of national housing policy', in Lowe, S. and Hughes, D. (eds) (1991) *A New Century of Social Housing?* Leicester: Leicester University Press.

Leather, P. and Morrison, T. (1997) *The State of UK Housing: A factfile on dwelling conditions*. York: Joseph Rowntree Foundation.

Lund, B. (1996) *Housing Problems and Housing Policy*. Social Policy in Britain Series. London: Longman.

Malpass, P. and Murie, A. (1999) *Housing Policy and Practice*. Fifth edition. London: Macmillan.

Marsh, A. and Mullins, D. (eds) (1998) *Housing and Public Policy: Citizenship, choice and control*. Buckingham: Open University.

Morris, J. (1990) *Our Homes our Rights: Housing independent living and physically disabled people*. London: Shelter.

Morris, J. and Winn, M. (1990) *Housing and Social Inequality*. London: Hilary Shipman.

National Federation of Housing Associations (1985) *Inquiry into British Housing 1st Report*. (2nd Report 1991). London: NFHA.

National Housing Forum (1997) *Living Places: Sustainable homes, sustainable communities*. London: NHF.

Oatley, N. (1998) *Cities, Economic Competition and Urban Policy*. London: Paul Chapman.

Pearl, M. (1997) *Social Housing Management: A critical appraisal of housing practice*. London: Macmillan.

Ravetz, A. with Turkington, R. (1995) *The Place of Home: English domestic environments, 1914–2000*. London: E and FN Spon.

Saunders, P. (1990) *A Nation of Home Owners*. London: Unwin Hyman.

Shelter (1998) *Access Denied*. London: Shelter.

Social Exclusion Unit (1998) *Bringing Britain Together: A national strategy for neighbourhood renewal*. Cmnd 4045. London: Cabinet Office.

Stephens, M. (1997) 'The windfall wars', in Goodwin, J. and Grant, C. (eds) (1997) *Built to Last? Reflections on British Housing Policy*. Second edition. London: *Roof* Magazine.

Thompson, K., Phelan, M., Strathdee, G. and Shiress, D. (1995) *Mental Health Care: A guide for housing workers.* London: The Mental Health Foundation

Wilcox, S. (1997) *Housing Finance Review 1997/98.* York: Joseph Rowntree Foundation.

Wilcox, S. (1998) *Housing Finance Review (1998/99).* York: Joseph Rowntree Foundation.

Williams, P (ed.) (1997) *Directions in Housing Policy: Towards sustainable housing policies in the UK.* London: Paul Chapman Publishing.

LIST OF THE MAIN UK HOUSING AGENCIES AND ORGANIZATIONS

Care and Repair The national co-ordinating body for home improvement agencies which was established in 1987 to provide low-income owner-occupiers with practical help with repairs, improvements and adaptations.

Chartered Institute of Housing (CIH) The professional body for housing officers and rent officers, which publishes two housing journals, *Inside Housing* (weekly) and *Housing* (monthly) as well as commissioning training materials and other publications.

Council of Mortgage Lenders (CML) The trade body for the mortgage lending industry.

Department of Environment, Transport and the Regions (DETR) The government department responsible for housing. Prior to the 1997 Labour government, the Department of the Environment (DOE) was responsible for housing.

Department of Health (DOH) The government department responsible for health issues.

Department of Social Security (DSS) The government department responsible for pensions and means-tested and non-means-tested welfare benefits

Housing Corporation (HC) Non-departmental public body that registers, regulates, funds and commissions research for Registered Social Landlords.

Housing Inspectorate (HI) Set up in 1999 within the Audit Commission as part of the Best Value regime. The inspectorate has a remit to monitor local authorities' Best Value programmes.

Joseph Rowntree Foundation (JRF) UK's largest independent research charity, providing grants for innovative development research and good practice in the fields of housing, social policy, social care and disability.

National Housing Federation (NHF) Represents the interests and concerns of Registered Social Landlords. The NHF undertakes research and provides an advisory function for its members.

Northern Ireland Housing Executive (NIHE) Set up in 1971 to manage local authority housing in Northern Ireland.

Registered Social Landlords (RSLs) This term was introduced in the 1996 Housing Act and includes housing associations, local housing companies and housing societies which are registered with the Housing Corporation.

Social Exclusion Unit (SEU) Set up by the 1997 Labour government to co-ordinate government programmes across education, social services, the police, the voluntary sector and housing.

Scottish Homes Established in 1989 to oversee housing association and housing co-operative activity in Scotland.

Scottish Office Deals with local authorities in Scotland and administers Scottish housing legislation.

Tai Cymru (Housing for Wales) Established in 1989 to take over the regulation of housing associations in Wales.

LIST OF ABBREVIATIONS

AIDS Acquired Immune Deficiency Syndrome
BES Business Expansion Scheme
BTEC Business Education Training Council
CIH Chartered Institute of Housing
CITB Construction Industry Training Board
CCT Compulsory Competitive Tendering
CRE Commission for Racial Equality
DETR Department of Environment, Transport and the Regions
DLO Direct Labour Organisation
DOE Department of the Environment
EA Estate Action
EMB Estate Management Board
ERCF Estate Renewal Challenge Fund
GIA General Improvement Area
GP General Practitioner
GRO Grants for Rent and Ownership
HA Housing Association
HAMA Housing Associations as Managing Agent
HARCA Housing and Regeneration Community Association
HATs Housing Actions Trusts
HC Housing Corporation
HITs Housing Investment Trusts
HMOs Houses in Multiple Occupation
ISA Individual Savings Account
IT Information Technology
LSVT Large-Scale Voluntary Transfers
MIRAS Mortgage Interest Relief at Source

NFHA National Federation of Housing Associations, latterly changed to NHF: National Housing Federation
NHF National Housing Federation
NHS National Health Service
NIHE Northern Ireland Housing Executive
NVQ National Vocational Qualification
PEP Personal Equity Plan, Priority Estate Project
PFA2000 People for Action 2000
PFI Private Finance Initiative
PPI Published Performance Indicator
RICS Royal Institute of Chartered Surveyors
RSL Registered Social Landlord
RTB Right to Buy
SNU Safe Neighbourhoods Unit
SRB Single Regeneration Budget
SVQ Scottish Vocational Qualification
TA Tenants Association
TB Tuberculosis
TPAS Tenant Participation Advisory Service
TMC Tenant Management Co-operative
TMO Tenant Management Organization
VCT Voluntary Competitive Tendering

SOME USEFUL INTERNET SITES

Housing and Social Policy Research

http://www.jrf.org.uk/
The first stop you should make when surfing the net is the Joseph Rowntree Foundation site. There is an archive of housing and housing-related research to make your mouth water, served up in a user-friendly way.

http://www.york.ac.uk/inst/chp
The Centre for Housing Policy at York is another easy-to-navigate site, with concise summaries of past research and commentary on on-going projects.

http://www.gla.ac.uk/Inter/CHRUS/
Glasgow University Centre for Housing Research and Urban Studies also has summaries of a wide range of relevant research. It not very user friendly, but it is worth the effort if you are a serious researcher.

http://www.london-research.gov.uk
The London Housing Research Centre carries out research and publishes regular bulletins and reports, mainly about London but a lot of the material is also of general interest.

Academic and professional journals

http://www.carfax.co.uk/
Housing Studies is the site of the heavyweight of housing journals. The site is well set out and provides an archive of past article titles, should you wish to pursue your studies in depth. The articles range from the extremely theoretical to those concerned with practice, but looked at from an academic viewpoint. Within the website, Housing Studies is located in the section on Journal information under the heading Geography, Planning and Development Journals.

The following three social housing publication sites are quite similar, each providing up-to-date housing news and a web version of the current issue of the magazine. However, Housing Today wins out over the other two because of its database search facility.

Inside Housing   http://www.atlas.co.uk/inside/

Housing Today   http://www.housingtoday.org.uk

Roof Magazine   http://www.shelter.org.uk/roof.html

Government, central and local

http://www.open.gov.uk
The main government site contains a useful organizational index which provides details of the individual sites of all central and local government departments.

DETR Home page   **http://www.detr.gov.uk/**

DETR Housing page   **http://www.housing.detr.gov.uk**

Without a doubt, the DETR site is a must for those studying housing. It is easy to navigate and has its own search engine. It contains a wealth of data, reports and consultative documents. It also has excellent links.

http://www.demon.co.uk/hcorp

While the Housing Corporation has a site, it has been out of action for some considerable time (as at March 1999), which is a pity since the corporation has such a key role in housing provision in this country and is destined to play an even bigger one. Watch this space!

http://www.lga.gov.uk/

The Local Government Association site contains a wealth of up-to-the-minute news, comment and information, responses to government proposals and details of initiatives it is undertaking. Like the DETR site, this is one you should always make a point of visiting.

Housing organizations

Most housing organizations have their own websites, but their quality and usefulness is variable. Below are the sites of a number of the better-known organizations: Shelter, TPAS, NHF, the Federation of Master Builders and the Building and Social Housing Foundation. Based in Coalville Leicestershire, the foundation maintains an active commitment to researching the possibilities for sustainable housing.

Shelter	**http://www.shelter.org.uk/main.html**
TPAS	**http://www.tpas.org.uk/**
NHF	**http://www.housing.org.uk**
FMB	**http://www.fmb.org.uk**
BSHF	**http://www.bshf.org.**

Housing link sites

Finally, here are two sites that provide links to a wide variety of housing-related sites on the net.

Housing Resource Guide	**http://www.housinguk.org**
General Housing Internet Resources	**http://www.housingnet.co.uk**

Index

165